Abundant Health

How to achieve your health potential

Insight from 29 dynamic health professionals

Cyndi O'Meara

CHANGING HABITS

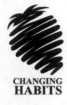

CHANGING HABITS

Abundant Health: How to Achieve Your Health Potential
Insight from 29 Dynamic Health Professionals

Published by Changing Habits www.changinghabits.com.au
PO Box 104 Mooloolaba QLD 4557 Australia

Editor: Suzanne Dean, Proof It Please
Project Manager: Carla Francis
Graphic Design: Holly Odgers, Allure Creative www.allurecreative.com.au
Cover Photos: Dreamstime and Stefan Postles www.stefanpostles.com.au
Printed in China by Everbest Printing Co.

Cataloguing in Publication Data:
O'Meara, Cyndi.
Abundant Health
ISBN 978-0-9752456-2-0
1. Health 2. Chiropractic 3. Nutrition

Disclaimer
Abundant Health is a new way of thinking about health. No responsibility is accepted by the authors or publisher for health care decisions made by readers. It is not a substitute for consulting your chosen health care professional. Always check with your health care professional.

DEDICATION

To all the wonderful contributors of
Abundant Health *who have made this project an
amazing journey of cooperation, sharing and giving.
Your dedication to helping people achieve physical,
mental and social wellbeing and health is to be
applauded by all you help and all you will help.*

Cyndi O'Meara

Contents

Foreword

During my twenty-five years in the field of health care I've written books, been interviewed by various members of the media and conducted seminars and educational programs for my clients, and working with people from many countries and learning from their expertise has strengthened my understanding of the importance of the vital truth in health. Since meeting Cyndi O'Meara I've developed great respect for her leadership in teaching people to care for themselves, so when Cyndi shared her vision to bring together a number of health professionals committed to educating people on a different way of looking at health, I knew it was an idea long overdue. This book is the result of that vision.

You are about to be faced with a challenge. In this book your most cherished ideas about health might be stomped on. Like a turbulent ride at a fun park, you will no doubt experience the stomach drop, and the pull, but stay in your seat – you will arrive safely at your destination, but having had a whole new experience. What you learn here could change your life.

Over the last few decades there has been a rise in people's awareness regarding their health as society has gradually begun to redefine health and where it comes from. People all over the world have begun questioning whether a particular pill, potion or procedure will be their best option or whether there is a different (even better) way. The idea of health coming to us is outdated. The future is here and it belongs to the person who understands that health is generated from within via their communication system – the nerve system. The chiropractic profession is at the forefront of this change as people source a different way and become empowered to change their lives.

This book describes a seismic worldwide shift. We are moving away from a society where our health care comes to us only via allopathic means. We are learning the value of a self-empowered understanding that health is created from within. Abundant Health is for anyone who is looking to move beyond the allopathic approach and acknowledge the innate intelligence that lives within each of us.

The stories in this book are about mothers, children, fathers, families, individuals and professionals coming to the realisation that there is another way to express health and in so doing are adding to this big shift. You will be exposed to the two different approaches to health care; you will read how the human body will function at optimum levels given no interference; you will learn why the first step in transforming your health is to transform your view of health, and you'll be provided with some steps to do this.

In *Abundant Health* you will read about those who have decided to live differently and be touched by the stories of chiropractors who have seen changes that have taken place faster than you think is possible, with less work than you would think possible. This book is all about making adjustments to the way you think and act, making it easier to create and express all the health you want, faster and easier than you could imagine.

And yes, there is a warning! You will find ideas in this book that are contrary and challenging to what you've been taught and to the beliefs that currently form the foundation of your actions. This material may make you uncomfortable but give yourself space to patiently and carefully consider the suggestions. Don't dismiss the ideas or the stories, for as you explore them you will see incredible opportunities to transform your life.

The people in these stories have chosen chiropractic for a reason. They've chosen to take responsibility for their health, knowing that a body clear of interference to its internal communication system is capable of changing and healing. They've chosen to do their life differently. I simply encourage you to read the contributions in this book, having made a decision that you will give the ideas room to develop in your own interpretation of health.

You will learn where health comes from, how to get it, and, most importantly, how to keep it. You will learn how magnificent you are. You will learn to trust your body.

Dr Sarah Farrant, DC
DC, Gen Sci, Grad Dip Psych, BA Phys Ed

CHAPTER 1

*"What lies behind us and what lies before us
are tiny matters compared to what lies within us"*

Ralph Waldo Emerson

Vitalism or Mechanism – It's Your Choice

By Sarah Farrant

The time was the 1800s. The industrial revolution was well underway. Factories were ablaze with smoking chimney stacks and people were certainly optimistic about their futures. In Davenport, Iowa, a little town on the Mississippi, boats were delivering cargo and picking up material to take elsewhere. In this bustling town, a discovery was about to emerge; a discovery that would change the direction of health care in the immediate present and foreseeable future. A discovery so great that people's lives would change as a result. Some would embrace and integrate this new understanding while others would be challenged and threatened and as a result attempt to stop the spread of this vital truth.

A young gentleman by the name of Daniel David Palmer (later to become known as "DD") had an office in the Ryan building in downtown Davenport. He was working as a magnetic healer at the time and was about to become the discoverer and founder of one of the world's best-kept secrets. Rev. Samuel Weed had been seeing DD Palmer for his exceptional magnetic healing and it was he who gave DD the name for the work he was doing – "CHIROPRACTIC" – derived from Greek root words meaning "done by hand."

DD went on to share the message of chiropractic in many ways. He became the first person to write about the connection between nerve system interference and the functioning of the human body. DD Palmer said, "Chiropractic was founded on tone ... the sole purpose of chiropractic is to reunite man the physical with man the spiritual."

From the early 1900s, both the chiropractic (vitalistic) and the medical (mechanistic) models of health have become more prominent, each with their own unique message to share – the medical model based on an understanding that the body requires help from the outside and the chiropractic model based on an understanding that your body has within it everything required to adapt, heal and grow.

I grew up in a mechanistic household when it came to health. I would cough, be wrapped in a blanket, bundled in the car and up to my uncle's, our family medical doctor, for the once over and a prescription. But I also grew up with a father who taught me about a different model: a vitalistic model. Dad didn't demonstrate it in health but he did in his line of work, which was stock broking and financial planning. He used to give presentations to large numbers of people and I would attend, listening to him and the messages he would share. At the age of seven he taught me there was a grander picture, a designed order to our life. He knelt down in front of me, looked me in the eye and, with his pointed finger, he so lovingly tapped over my heart and said:

> *"Sarah you have all the answers inside of you.*
> *All you have to do is ask the question and be*
> *prepared to hear the answer."*

Those sentences changed my life. When I was driving with Mum in the car at the age of ten up to my uncle's to see someone, to get something, to take something away, I found myself remembering those words Dad told me. I turned to Mum and said, "He's just going to give me another prescription for Amoxcil but all I need to do is rest."

And sure enough, that day changed my life. I rejected the medication placed on the kitchen bench by Mum when we returned home and I went around to my room and rested. I trusted that I knew what to do. Rarely from that day forth did I tell Mum or Dad of a sign or symptom I might have been having – what I now call a "health expression."

It wasn't until I got to Palmer College of Chiropractic in Davenport, Iowa, where the profession began, that I heard a word that resonated so deep with my being, a word so true for me. It was during my first philosophy class and the teacher said "Vitalism". I left that day with many illusions about health and life broken and headed straight to the library, went to the internet and looked up everything on vitalism. When I read the material I knew it was vitalism my dad had been teaching me in life and wealth. And at the age of ten, when I decided to take responsibility and listen to my body and hear the message, I knew that I had taken this understanding of vitalism Dad had taught me about wealth and was applying it to my health. Now I was able to place a word on it. My vision, since the launch of my award-winning book *The Vital Truth*®, has and will continue to be "to share vitalistic philosophy with the world and how it relates to health for the purpose of changing the health consciousness of individuals, families, communities, cities, states, nations and the world; to inspire a desire in others to do their life differently; to ask different questions."

I now sing the praises of vitalism and chiropractic, which is the largest health care profession in the world using no drugs or surgery, only your body's innate ability to heal, adapt and change. For it's not about the back or the crack! It is about neurological integrity, adaptation and potential – your life potential.

You're probably wondering at this point, "What is the major difference between mechanism and vitalism? Well ...

The mechanist and the vitalist have been arguing with each other for well over 2500 years about what actually constitutes health and disease and what signs and symptoms represent. Vitalism respects the structure and function of living things while at the same time recognising and acknowledging an "innate intelligence" that designed and keeps the whole working at its optimum.

The mechanistic theory views the smallest components of the physical body's structure as building blocks. These blocks are understood to make up the whole. This view, however, leaves no room for an innate intelligence, looking only at problems in isolation rather than in the complete interconnected form. The mechanistic approach maintains that the body is powerless to perform self-growth and healing, assuming a "fix it" mentality, and has the user take on a passive participant role. This assumption places a higher value on the educated mind than on a body that actually made itself.

Until 1932, the mechanistic view of health was widely accepted – then something astounding happened. Ernst Rutherford split the atom and discovered that "matter" was comprised mostly of "space". This seemingly empty space was actually a large amount of energy unable to be seen with the naked eye. It became obvious that energy played a critical role in keeping the atom together and in the process this brought vitalistic philosophy back into the limelight.

Since the 1950s, the mechanistic philosophy has wavered. Doctors who were once respected were now being questioned. The Baby Boomers questioned authority in the '60s, challenging everything from scientific thinking to health choices. The growth of mass media made spreading new values an easy process and today people are making informed choices about their philosophy, their values and their health care.

A chiropractor senses that it is not enough to understand the "building blocks". Chiropractors who understand vitalistic philosophy recognise that "something" – an essential energy – is responsible for organising the human body. Innately we keep the body functional using this energy and optimise the expression of it via the nerve system. This intelligence, this life force, this energy, is the difference between a corpse and a living body, and when the body has everything in balance, it is better able to express health to its fullest potential.

Vitalism acknowledges an innate intelligence that exists in us all – an intelligence that enables us to function without thought. Our innate intelligence, our life force, uses the nerve system – the master system of the body – to express itself. Our nerve system coordinates the "conversations", if you will, between all the systems, organs, tissues, cells, organelles, molecules, atoms, subatomic particles, vibrations, energy and light.

Vitalism brings a different approach to health care. The innate intelligence of the body which created it really *does* have the ability to heal it. What happens when we cut our finger? The body heals it. A whole chain of events takes place in just the right sequence, in just the right amounts and at just the right time in order for the platelet coagulation to take place at the site of the cut. Within the vitalistic model there is greater incentive to be the observer in one's ability to express health. This "way of life" philosophy enables us to check in with ourselves, to ask different questions, to awaken ourselves to our imbalances and to listen for the answers we require for our health and make choices accordingly.

A personal responsibility goes with this way of thinking for our health. I encourage each of you to investigate further the philosophy of vitalism and how it relates to your health. For those who are comfortable with this philosophy, acknowledge the internal wisdom of your body in its ability to heal itself. With this knowledge, people are making healthier choices, and chiropractic is playing a large and vital role.

CHAPTER 2

> *"It is not a question of whether man chooses to be guided by [philosophy]: he is not equipped to live without it."*
>
> Ayn Rand

A Healthy Philosophy

By Rosemary Folker

I was first introduced to the subject of philosophy when, as a mature student, I was studying psychology A-level. At the time I wondered what on earth philosophy had to do with psychology, but I soon came to realise that philosophy is interwoven with every subject. Philosophy is, in fact, interwoven with everything, with the very fabric of life, although many of us do not necessarily think of it affecting our own lives in particular.

So what is philosophy and what does it have to do with our health? Whether you choose to see a medical doctor or an alternative practitioner, does the philosophy of that discipline make any difference to your experience as a patient and, if so, in what way? I aim to show in this chapter that philosophy, our own and that of the discipline we're thinking of choosing, does make a difference when it comes to our health because it affects our whole experience as an individual. I would argue that chiropractic is, in fact, very different to medicine and it is the philosophy of chiropractic that makes that difference. How much your own philosophy of health ties in with that of chiropractic, will probably affect how you use it, either for short-term pain relief or as a long-term lifestyle choice.

First of all, it could be helpful to ask ourselves, "What is philosophy?" Quite literally, the term "philosophy" means "love of wisdom." In general terms, philosophy is an activity we undertake when we seek to understand fundamental truths about ourselves, the world in which we live and our relationship to each other and the world itself. Philosophy, as an academic discipline, raises some of the deepest and widest questions there are and looks for answers through rational argument and logical reasoning. Philosophy is traditionally divided into the study of major areas such as the theory of reality, knowledge, ethics (moral values), politics and aesthetics (the theory of beauty and art).

We could sum up philosophy as studying "the fundamental nature of existence, of man, and of man's relationship to existence. ... In the realm of cognition, the special sciences are the trees, but philosophy is the soil, which makes the forest possible." Ayn Rand, *Philosophy, Who Needs It* (p. 2).

In terms of our own lives, philosophy could be seen as an integrated system of ideas about human nature and the nature of the reality we live in.

> *It is a guide for living, because the issues it addresses are basic and pervasive, determining the course we take in life and how we treat other people.*

According to novelist and philosopher Ayn Rand, we don't have a choice as to whether we have a philosophy, "but only which philosophy to have", and whether our philosophy "will be conscious, explicit, logical, and therefore practical – or random, unidentified, contradictory, and therefore lethal".

So now we know what philosophy is, we can ask, what does it have to do with our health? If we take heed of Ayn Rand's words, it would seem wise to actively choose our philosophy in the different areas of our lives, and no more so than when it comes to our health. When we've chosen, it would then seem reasonable to find a health discipline whose philosophy is congruent with our own. As we've said, philosophy is a guide for living; it determines our beliefs and values, which in turn determine the actions we take. Likewise, the philosophy of a health discipline determines the beliefs and values to which that discipline subscribes, which in turn tends to dictate the actions taken within that discipline. As the philosophy of chiropractic is different to the philosophy of medicine, your experience in a chiropractic office will probably be quite different to your experience in a medical doctor's office.

> *However, because in our society we have grown up with one dominant model of health, that is a medical model, we often don't realise that there are other choices we can make.*

In my experience of managing a chiropractic office, many people seem to end up consulting a chiropractor having been referred by a family member or friend. Some have tried the medical route without success, or hear about chiropractic and choose it as an alternative or, perhaps, a last resort. This is fine as far as it goes; however, an active health choice is surely more beneficial than simply choosing, without question or knowledge, what we've grown up with. Being consciously aware of our own philosophy on health would be a start in helping to guide the choices we make.

Given this, then, what is the philosophy of chiropractic and how will it impact your health and your experience as a patient? Firstly, we need to understand the ways chiropractic can be seen as different to medicine.

Bill Esteb, a well-known advocate of chiropractic who lectures to chiropractors around the world on the patient's point of view, makes the following major and useful distinctions between the two health disciplines. Chiropractic is nerve based; that is, chiropractors are concerned with whether our nerves and our nervous system are being compromised in any way; whereas medicine is blood based; it is concerned with whether our blood is normal or not, within certain test ranges. Also, chiropractic looks to correct the cause of a problem whereas medicine, by and large, tends to treat symptoms. This is fundamental in chiropractic, which sees treating symptoms rather than the cause as rather like painting over the oil warning light in your car. The oil is still low but all would seem fine because you can no longer see the light. Another distinction is that chiropractic concerns itself with the whole person, whereas medicine is more concerned with the body as parts; for example, "the appendicitis in bed five". Chiropractors make adjustments to the body, whereas medicine tends to rely on drugs or surgery. Surgery often involves removing organs, whereas chiropractic is about reviving them. Lastly, but importantly, chiropractic is seen as natural and working with the body, whereas medicine, one could argue, is artificial and, with that, more risky.

Chiropractic produces positive effects rather than *side* effects, as is often the case with drugs, and helps the immune system to the extent that many chiropractic patients report that they suffer fewer colds and flu viruses because their bodies are more able to resist germs. Medicine, however, tends to be threatened by germs and sees the body as succumbing to them rather than being able to resist them.

Now, before we talk about the philosophy of chiropractic, we should be aware that there has been, and still is, controversy over some of the statements above. Detractors and skeptics of chiropractic argue that it is not necessarily that effective, safe or beneficial to the body as a whole. Unfortunately, more research is done into medicine than chiropractic because medical research tends to be funded by drug companies, who have plentiful funds, whereas chiropractic, along with other natural disciplines, does not have that advantage. Therefore, chiropractic research is slow and much of the data is to be found in the form of actual case studies and patient's stories or anecdotes when assessing the claims of chiropractic. Until more research can be done, we are mostly reliant upon this. However, having said that, we cannot totally rely on science either, in whatever matter that's being investigated, because no truth is absolute. Truth is only as good as the information we have at any one time.

Throughout history, scientists have pronounced truths in various matters only to be found wrong later or, what they found be true at the time has had to be revised in the light of the accumulation of new information. This still happens. A basic, easy example, if an old one, is that at one time it was thought that the earth was flat, only to be corrected by Copernicus and Galileo whose revolutionary discovery overturned this accepted truth. With regard to medicine, which is often thought of as more scientifically based, the same point applies. Currently accepted medical ideas may not necessarily be true and could be overturned to make way for new ideas in the future. I think it's worth being aware of this and ...

> ... *not be tempted to revere medicine without question,*
> *only to reject other health disciplines, also without question.*

Having looked then, at the ways in which chiropractic can be viewed as being different to medicine, we come to the philosophy that chiropractic holds that all living things are maintained by innate intelligence, sometimes called "life force". We could think of this intelligence as the inner wisdom of the body which guides all automatic functions and regulates the body, continually adapting it to the environment so it stays healthy. Your body knows exactly what it needs and how to adapt to the environment in order to function best. We don't need to think, for example, how to digest food, eliminate waste, heal a cut or fight infections. This happens automatically, courtesy of our innate intelligence. In other words, your body is self-regulating and self-healing with health being viewed as coming from within. This is the concept of Vitalism. Furthermore, the philosophy of chiropractic holds that innate intelligence is an expression of universal intelligence, that is to say there is an intelligent order to the universe, a level of organisation to it, or a grand design. Whether we choose to believe that such a level of order must have required some sort of grand designer or creator (God?), and some people do believe this, or whether it is "the existing principle of an organising principle manifesting itself" (Ian Coulter, *Chiropractic A Philosophy for Alternative Health Care*, p.39) is up to you to ponder. You wouldn't be alone, as it is a major philosophical question in itself.

Holism, another philosophical concept, is the idea that the whole is greater than the sum of its parts. In chiropractic, your whole being is considered in terms of your physical, mental and spiritual health and many chiropractors will include advice on nutrition, exercise, postural and stress management. Some chiropractic techniques also deal with emotional issues.

There is also the concept of neural supremacy, which, in effect, says that all organs, tissues and cells are controlled and regulated by the nervous system. In other words, the nervous system coordinates all body parts and functions, sending messages in the form of electrical impulses from your brain to all your cells. Chiropractors are concerned with removing any interference to these messages getting through.

Another philosophical belief in chiropractic is the idea of Conservatism or, because they believe in the body's ability to heal itself, it follows that care should be the least invasive and the idea that "less is more" is important. Chiropractic adjustments are carefully administered and work with the body rather than against it, as drugs can do (Dean Black, *Health at the Crossroads*).

Finally, the moral philosophy of Humanism, which is concerned with human beings being treated with dignity, equality and caring, is vital to your experience when consulting any health professional and should be evident no more so than in a chiropractic office. Humanism, which says that these rights cannot be given up or taken away, is a central concept in chiropractic. Ian Coulter points to a study, which found that chiropractors actively encourage and empower their patients to participate in their care by explaining their health concerns to them and by educating them about chiropractic and how it relates to their health. He calls it "co-operative care, with the patients as partners", taking responsibility for their own health. In addition, many chiropractors try to create a warm and friendly environment, seeing this, along with customer service, as important.

Whether you choose to see a medical doctor or a chiropractor, does the philosophy of that discipline make any difference to your experience as a patient and, if so, in what way? Well, we can see from above that the answer is a definite yes. To sum it up, the concepts above, and whether they are evident and/or important in any health discipline of your choosing, will dictate your treatment regimen, how your body is viewed and whether your lifestyle is seen as an important factor in your decline in health and also your recovery. It will also affect how invasive your care may be and whether it works in harmony with your body or not and, finally, how you are treated as a person. Of course, we are all different in our views and needs and you have to decide what concepts are important to you as a health consumer or, as we would think of it in chiropractic, a health participant! The extent to which you take on the philosophy of chiropractic in your quest for health will also affect how you wish to use it: as a choice for pain relief, which chiropractic is good at, or whether you take it further and use chiropractic as a lifestyle choice. It is totally up to you. It's your body, your life and your choice.

CHAPTER 3

*"There is no passion to be found playing small – in settling
for a life that is less than the one you are capable of living."*

Nelson Mandela

A New Way to Health is Born

By Jennifer Layton

The first emergence of chiropractic as we know it was September 1895, in Davenport, Iowa, when a man's hearing loss was returned to normal by having his spine adjusted by a Mr Daniel David Palmer. However, looking through history, he was not the first to realise the importance of the spine to health.

Much earlier than this, knowledge of the spine as a causative agent in pain and disease had been apparent, for example, to the Greek physician and teacher you may have heard of called Hippocrates (460 to 375 BC). He knew the importance of the spine to staying healthy, even writing two books on the topic. The essence of chiropractic was captured in his teaching when he said, "Get the knowledge of the spine, for it is the requisite for many diseases." Hippocrates was also reported to have stressed to his students that it is nature that does the healing and the doctor only removes obstructions to that healing, which is what chiropractors are informing their patients to this day.

Some 200 years later, the Latin physician Galen (200 to 130 BC) was the first to teach the relationships and positions of the spine, and when teaching his students about the nerve system, emphasised the importance of it to maintaining health.

But long before this, spinal manipulation had been done by the Ancient Egyptians, recorded with hieroglyphics on ancient papyrus; and even much earlier again, spinal manipulation had been noted by the ancient Chinese.

Which brings us back to Davenport, Iowa, in September 1895. This latter part of the 19th century was a real time of change and of growing awareness in science and technology. Already the period had provided people with steamboats and the railroad and machines for other tasks. Conventional medicine at this time was looking for a change from the use of the addictive morphine and the toxic mercury in tackling a disease to less harmful solutions for the removal of symptoms, which led to the growing use by the public of homeopathy, magnetic healing and osteopathy as solutions with fewer side-effects. By the mid-1800s, medical schools were cheap and plentiful, producing an over-supply of physicians and therefore driving the physicians' incomes down. Their answer to this was to form a medical association to raise the standard of education and by doing so, limiting the number of new physicians and protecting their incomes. This then set the scene for the first chiropractic adjustment.

Now back to our man DD Palmer who was born in Canada in 1845, a character with a big personality and an even bigger beard. He was working as a magnetic healer, which was a popular therapy at the time, along with the newly developed fields of homeopathy and osteopathy. Whilst working late one night in his magnetic healing office, he observed that the building's janitor failed to hear the noise of a passing fire truck. This janitor, a Mr Harvey Lillard, had been deaf for seventeen years following a bending injury in which he had damaged his upper back, even saying he heard a popping sound at the time of the injury.

On noting this, DD used his knowledge of the spine and applied pressure to the injury site. After two such treatments, Mr Lillard's hearing had returned. Buoyed by this success, DD used this new technique for his patients and recorded even more successes. His new discovery now needed a name, so he asked his client and friend, the Rev Samuel Weed, who had been a student of language, to come up with a name for this new discovery. That suggestion was, of course, *chiropractic*, which is from the Greek "cheiros praktikos" meaning "done by hand". DD recognised that the body had a natural state of health and therefore sickness is a departure from this natural state by some sort of interference in the body's own healing abilities. Gaining a reputation as a healer who produced results, DD then set up the Palmer School of Chiropractic, which is still going strong today under the title of Palmer College of Chiropractic.

In 1906, DD's son, BJ Palmer, took over the reins (which he held until his death in 1961) and developed the profession and the study of chiropractic. He was only a youngster of 20 when he took command of the chiropractic school and so grew the same big beard as his dad to appear older. The college grew, partly due to the benefits paid to war veterans who could then afford to study and were in search of a career, so they studied at this or one of the many other chiropractic schools that flourished at the time. By the early 1920s there were more than 80 chiropractic schools in the USA; but then the veterans' benefits expired and many schools closed. Following this, though, at the remaining schools, education content increased with an enhanced stress on diagnosis. By the 1930s there was a push to make the course four years long.

BJ was quite an innovator and an early adaptor of new technology. He was one of the first to use x-rays for visualising the spine and then teaching this to his students. He called it "spinography" and this was in 1910, before the medical profession made use of the technology. He started a radio station in Davenport in 1922, called WOC (standing for World of Chiropractic) and, noticing his potential for greater things, employed an up-and-coming young star named Ronald Reagan.

Chiropractic still suffered its hardships during its development, mostly through the threat of chiropractors being sent to prison for "practising medicine without a licence", a fate that was in store for hundreds of chiropractors, including our friend DD Palmer who was jailed in 1906 for six months. One poor fellow was arrested twelve times and jailed four times, holding the record for the most jailed chiropractor. The search for chiropractors to be jailed was enforced by the state medical boards, sending in plain-clothed policemen to gather evidence. However, it was seen that patients rarely agreed to testify against their chiropractor.

Through the years, though, chiropractic gained in popularity as the results spoke for themselves, although the profession was lacking in research. This was attended to and research became a serious pursuit from the 1970s, with journals, both chiropractic and medical, publishing research that backed the results patients were experiencing and supporting the theories of DD and BJ Palmer with regard to the healing power of the chiropractic adjustment. Through this period of the 1970s, admission requirements were tightened at colleges, and the profession is now formally regulated in over 60 countries.

Currently there are more than thirty accredited institutions teaching chiropractic throughout the world, awarding a bachelor's degree or higher to the graduates. Chiropractors learn many different techniques to adjust their patient's spines, with over 100 in existence, and all work and are effective. Some techniques are old, similar to the way DD Palmer adjusted the spine of Harvey Lillard, and some techniques are much newer. Some use the hand to deliver an adjustment, and some use a special table, or an adjusting instrument, or the force of gravity. But the important thing to remember is, no matter which technique is used, they all have benefits.

From these beginnings, chiropractic has grown and is now the third largest health profession in the world, behind medicine and dentistry.

CHAPTER 4

"It's not what you are that holds you back;
it's what you think you are not."

Denis Waitley

Inspiring Change

By Paula Moore

We all want to be healthy and happy. We desire more vitality, more energy, more attractiveness and as we get older we spend more time thinking about our health. Often when we think of health we think of how we would like to change our current state of health – from smoking to not smoking, from being large to being thin, from not exercising to exercising, or from eating junk food to eating "healthy" food. Before we consider becoming healthier, I suggest that we first need a new view of health, a paradigm shift, a new possibility for our health and ourselves.

I created the possibility of *living naturally* when I first began studying chiropractic at the age of twenty-eight. I had started having daily headaches in my early twenties, a short while after a minor road traffic accident. At that time I thought nothing about taking aspirin several times a week. Aspirin seemed to work, ridding me of my unwanted headache. When I had my first chiropractic adjustment years later, my headaches disappeared instantly. I was so amazed by this healing art that I decided to return to university as a mature student and study chiropractic.

About one year into my five-year degree, I had an epiphany, a total paradigm shift. I had met hundreds of happy, healthy individuals (chiropractic students, international chiropractic speakers, chiropractors and their families raised naturally and thriving). They all seemed to share one thing in common, an absolute passion for natural health and healing, and I knew then that this was my truth. It was crystal clear. I had woken up, and for the first time in my life I understood the meaning of health. I was forever transformed and it seemed to happen in an instant!

So now, almost fifteen years later, I can say that I have never been more inspired to enjoy a relatively natural life. I choose not to medicate, allowing my body to learn, strengthen and heal from illness. I enjoy the regular support I receive from my healing profession. I eat mostly good quality unadulterated organic food, and I exercise. My home is largely free of toxic chemicals (that means I save a lot of money on toiletries, lotions and potions) and I surround myself with healthy, like-minded individuals.

Changing our health is often about changing our behavior or changing the way we feel. This chapter is not, however, about changing our health or health habits in a familiar way. This chapter is about *transforming* our health. For distinction, let us say that "transformation" is a different experience of "change". We can use a simple example for clarity. Take a particular shape, a square. Now let's change that square. It becomes a rectangle or a triangle or a circle. Now take that same square and this time let's transform the square. It becomes a cube. It becomes more of itself. It has transformed.

When you change, you may lose weight, start exercising or alter your eating habits. When you transform, you actually expand (not physically) and with expansion your patterns of behavior and feelings alter and you become more of yourself. Transformation of health has you throw out the old model (your past relationship to health) and invent something that was not there before.

Transforming your health may feel disruptive but with transformation you cannot help but succeed. We have a lot of control over our actions but relatively little control over our feelings. With transformation, for instance, you may find that you choose to exercise even though you don't feel like exercising.

So what is currently available for us in the world of health? It would be fair to say that western health care providers largely believe that pain and symptoms are undesirable, so the eradication of symptoms and disease is at the forefront of modern medicine. What if pain, disease and illness had a purpose? What if we considered pain, disease and illness a necessary part of health? What if our pain, disease and illness allow our body to strengthen its inborn ability to heal? Now if that were true (and I am suggesting that it is) we could transform our view of health by accepting the ways things already are.

We could begin with an acceptance of our current state of health at this very moment in time. By acceptance, I don't mean resignation. Acceptance of the reality of our circumstances *can* provide freedom, and perhaps a clean slate on which to begin a new journey, one I call "being healthy".

If you are upset about your current state of health, then it is time to get excited. Your being upset suggests that you are committed to your health. If you were not committed you would not be upset. The bigger your upset, the bigger your commitment. If you are committed to nothing, then you have no upset. You would not argue and get upset with your family if you were not committed to having good relationships with them. Your degree of upset is proportional to your degree of commitment. If you are upset about your weight, a recent medical diagnosis, your lack of energy, or your eating habits, then it is time to get excited because you are committed to having better health.

In England, and in other western countries, a quarter of all adults (age 16 and older) are obese.[1] We know more about obesity, diet and nutrition than ever before – there are 20,000 diet books currently available on Amazon. This seems to suggest that simply learning or knowing more about our current state of health doesn't necessarily change our health behavior, so it may be time to transform our view of health.

The first step in transforming your health is to transform your view of health by declaring a commitment to *being in health*. As I said before, if you are upset with your current state of health, then you can be sure you are committed to your health. This is the perfect place to begin.

The second step in transforming your health is to create a new possibility for your health. Now let's be clear – you all possess health, all of you! It may not be a health expression with which you feel happy but, nonetheless, it is what it is at this moment and there is only today, this minute, the present, to begin your transformation. You can choose right now to transform your health and to invent a new possibility for your health that inspires you.

Your possibility is about your state of *being* and may look something like this:

> *I am creating the possibility of (you fill this in)*
> *for my health and my life.*

(Below are a few examples of possibilities you could choose. You may prefer to write your own.)

I am creating the possibility of living naturally for my health and my life.

I am creating the possibility of being vibrant for my health and my life.

I am creating the possibility of youthful energy for my health and my life.

I am creating the possibility of vitality and fun for my health and my life.

The third step in transforming your health is to choose a health care discipline that will support your health transformation. For me, that discipline is chiropractic (the world's third largest primary health care profession).[2] Chiropractors are primary health care physicians with a wholistic view of health. Chiropractors put forth that healing comes from the inside out, not from the outside in. In other words, most chiropractors believe that we are born with an innate ability to heal our bodies without need for external interference (namely drugs and surgery). Chiropractors accept that pain, disease and illness are a necessary part of the process of gaining and maintaining health. In a sense, pain and illness may be understood as the body's natural ability to communicate imbalance. Chiropractors understand that "health is a state of complete physical, mental and social wellbeing and not merely the absence of disease or infirmity".[3]

You may choose to leave step three out completely and go it alone and some of you may like the support of more than one discipline. Whatever way you choose to transform, be certain that your likelihood of success increases with the support of others.

So you have taken the first step and declared your commitment to your health (regardless of your current state of health). You have taken the second step and created a new possibility for your health that inspires you, and you have taken the third step in transforming your health by choosing a health care discipline to support your journey, which for many of you will be chiropractic.

The fourth and final step in transforming your health is to take action. This is usually the point at which many of us feel confronted. The secret to taking action is to have an action plan. Your action plan begins with your possibility. If you recall, I created the possibility of living naturally. To live naturally, I needed an action plan in which to measure my progress.

My action plan included living without the use of medication, eating mainly good quality organic food (where possible), exercising regularly and living in an environment with minimal toxic chemical exposure. Each action required mini action steps. For instance, changing the quality of food that I consumed had me take many actions over a period of weeks and months.

Some of the action steps I created for myself included:

- Fitting a carbon water filter onto my kitchen taps

- Finding an organic butcher

- Having an organic veggie box delivered

- Attending local farmers markets

The action steps need to be specific and attainable and you need to find some way to ensure that you will remember to take each action. I liked noting the actions into my monthly diary. Some of you may prefer to use a phone diary or a computer software program. Make it easy for yourself.

We all want to be healthy and happy. Perhaps your view of health has already started to shift and you are ready to transform your health starting now, this moment. Remember that transforming your health begins with transforming your view of health by declaring a commitment to being "in health". Share your commitment and it will begin to have a life of its own. Tell someone now; declare it! You don't have to wait for something to change. Begin this minute. Declare your commitment.

Now you've invented that new possibility for your health and your life, write it down, speak it, share it and get excited by it! If you are not yet excited you haven't chosen the right possibility for your health transformation.

Next, choose a health care discipline that will support your new possibility. Chiropractic is one of many wholistic approaches to health care and one I strongly recommend for your health transformation.

Finally, it is time to take action. Get an action plan down on paper. Put it in your diary, on your mirror, in your car, on your phone and on your computer. Live your new possibility through your experiences and stop worrying about whether or not you *feel* like being your possibility. *Be* your possibility because you are committed to your health and your life. When you slip off the wagon, jump straight back on and don't make it mean that you have failed. Just go back to step one and start again, and again and again if you have to, and before you know it you will awaken one morning to find that you have transformed your health and you will recognise this and what a glorious day it will be.[4]

CHAPTER 5

*"Anatomy is to physiology as geography is to
history; it describes the theatre of events."*

Jean François Fernel

(*De Naturali Parte Medicinae
Libri Septem* (1542), Ch. 1.)

Anatomy
of Health

By Neil Folker

I n order to know *how* to be healthy it's important to know what your body
does and how it works. To do *that* it really helps to have some knowledge of
how it's put together.

Now, there are *lots* of aspects to anatomy. A full edition of *Gray's Anatomy*
(*the* anatomy textbook) runs to nearly 1500 pages! What we're going to
concentrate on here are the parts that are most immediately relevant to
chiropractic and its effect on your health. As you may know, in terms of the
treatment carried out, chiropractors place great emphasis on your spine.
Let's see why.

The master control system in your whole body is your nervous system. This is
the system that runs the show. As stated in Guyton's physiology textbook (an
ultimate reference), it's your nervous system that governs *all* the processes in

your body and therefore is the aspect of your body that controls your health. It makes sense then to protect this "master" system. It so happens that your nerves are quite fragile and their function can be dramatically reduced by pressure on them, so your nervous system is protected by bone inside your skull and your spinal column. This serves to protect it from the rigours of daily activity fairly well. However, these nerves still have to exit from your spine to run to every part of your body, and this is where they can become irritated. Let's see how your spine is put together.

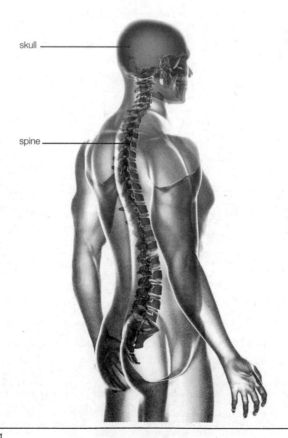

skull

spine

Figure 1

Your spinal column, i.e. the bony part (the spinal cord is the nerves part), is a marvel of engineering (it's not *a* backbone; it's many bones). It supports the weight of your upper body and allows a degree of flexibility and movement as well as protecting your spinal cord. There are gaps between the 26 bones of your spine and here the nerves exit your spine and branch off to supply every part of you. Your nervous system is so all-pervasive that if you could take away everything else and leave the nerves behind, you'd be there in such perfect detail that you'd be perfectly recognisable (although not as attractive, it's true to say). From the different levels of your spine, the nerves run to particular areas of your skin and particular muscles. There is a set pattern to this, like a map. Specific levels go to specific places. (See figure 2.)

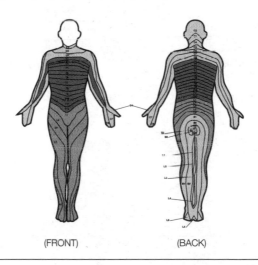

(FRONT)   (BACK)

Figure 2

So how is your spinal cord enclosed in your vertebrae (the bones in your spine)? Your vertebrae have a large, roughly cotton-reel-like part at the front and these are separated from the bones above and below by discs (more of those later). Then, at the back of the vertebrae is a part with the facet joints on it; these guide the movement. Between these two parts there is a canal (the aptly named spinal canal) that houses the spinal cord. (See figures 3 and 4.)

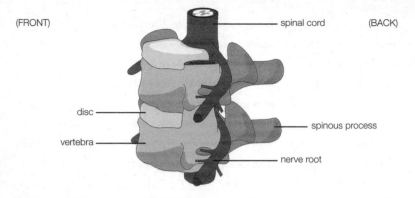

Figure 3

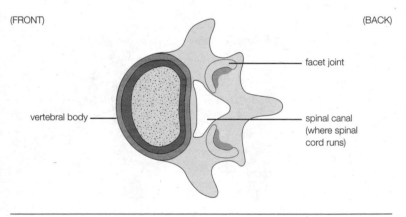

Figure 4

Let's look at the structure of your spine and nervous system from the top down. Starting with your brain inside your skull, this is very firmly attached inside. Even so, in the case of a violent blow or movement, the brain can move about in your head and be "bruised" (concussed – you have concussion). There is evidence that the bones of your skull normally move very slightly in a rhythm. This is thought to be tied in with the circulation of fluid around your nervous system and is treated with a variety of gentle chiropractic cranial techniques.

Below your skull is your top vertebra or Atlas. This bone is of prime importance as it can be thought of as the fine tuning on your balance and posture. It is also unique in that it's not fixed to the other vertebrae by a disc but rather sits like a ring on a peg that's part of the one below (the Axis). The Atlas can move differently and surrounds the brain stem itself. There are many chiropractic techniques that place great importance on this vertebra and its relative position. Problems here can have far-reaching effects on our nervous system. Below this, are the remaining top seven bones which comprise your cervical spine. These should form a curve which, when seen from the side, has a hollow at the back of your neck. They are often referred to as C1 to C7. Below these are the Thoracic vertebrae. Twelve in number, these have your ribs attached to them and are called T1 to T12 (or sometimes D1 to D12, D for dorsal, another word for thoracic). They should have an outward curve to them.

The bottom of your spine is your Lumbar spine. These five bones are larger than the others, as they support more weight. Here, once again, you should have a slight hollow in your back to follow the curve they make.

Underneath this is your pelvis. It's made up of three large bones: the triangular sacrum at the back and the two ilia (ilium is the singular) either side. These are joined together by the sacroiliac joints at the back (roughly where the little dimples are above your bottom either side) and the pubis symphysis at the front. The socket parts of the ball and socket-like hip joint are contained in the outer/lower part of each ilium. Your coccyx is, incidentally, the tiny piece of bone at the bottom tip of your sacrum. (For further reading see *Gray's Anatomy*, though be careful with your back – it's a bit on the heavy side!) All these bones are held together by the muscles (see below) and the ligaments. Ligaments are short inelastic "strings" that hold bones together and can shorten or tighten with lack of use or be overstrained in injuries.

The curves in your spine are very important and act like shock absorbers, or springs, to cushion us as we walk. We can lose these curves when our spine degenerates, or in response to chronic strain. They can also be lost, or distorted, in cases of acute strain or injury. The curves also enable us to move well. Look at how flexible, and curved, a flamingo's neck is!

So, your spine has to be able to bend, twist, flex and stretch in many directions, all the while protecting your nervous system. By and large, it does a good job of this but the nerves run close to the discs and facet joints between the vertebrae and they can be chafed or irritated here, often at their exit of the spine between the vertebrae. In chiropractic this is often referred to as a subluxation. That "map" we mentioned earlier, can help us pin down where a nerve is compromised in this way.

Inside your spine, the nerves all branch off at each level to run throughout your body. There are really a number of parts to your nervous system. The first is your central nervous system – your brain and spinal cord. The second is your peripheral nervous system, comprising all the nerves that run throughout your body and send messages to and from your brain. These control muscles and joints and carry feedback about touch, temperature, pressure, position etc. The other component of your nervous system is your autonomic nervous system. This does all the things you don't have to think about, millions of them! It runs all the "background" workings of your body ... your heart rate, kidney function, liver activity, digestion, immune system, blood pressure, blood sugar levels, all of it. All without you thinking about it, and this system can be irritated in just the same way as your peripheral nerves can. That map applies here too, with different levels of your spine giving the nerve supply to different organs in your body. These nerves carry "control" information to and from the brain and if these are affected, an organ may not work as it should.

We must also touch on the muscles that move our spine around. There are many varied shapes and sizes in your spine. Some run between just two vertebrae, whilst others are much larger and move your shoulder, arm, leg etc. Suffice it to say, that the tone (that is to say, the amount of tension or degree of contraction at rest) is critical. It must be within the normal range and be balanced left to right.

Strange though it may seem, we're not supremely well adapted for being upright. We battle gravity every day and don't help ourselves by overloading ourselves or flexing our spines in chairs for hours on end (let alone sitting in cars or at computers all day!). In the process of straining our spine, whether it be through, amongst other things, acute injury, overwork or being stuck in one position, these joints (discs and facets) can malfunction and nerve irritation or compression (subluxation) can result. Let's see how.

Next, discs.

> *Discs don't slip. I know it's a common phrase, and even medical doctors use it, but it's very misleading.*

The spinal discs are firmly anchored to the bones above and below them. A disc is like a cushion and consists of two parts. The outer part, the annulus or ring, is a circle of thick ligaments that runs in alternating spirals (think radial car tyre). Contained in the centre of this, like jam in a doughnut, is the nucleus, a toothpaste-like substance that is under pressure and acts as a shock absorber. (See figure 5.) If the disc is subjected to too many stresses and strains over time, the outer layers, the annulus, can break down and nucleus material can bulge outwards through the thinner layers. This is like the weakness in the wall of an old tyre, or a misshapen cushion. This is called a disc bulge. If the strain is severe enough, or prolonged enough, the annulus can break down entirely and the inner disc material spills out under pressure and becomes a ruptured or prolapsed disc. This is very much like the jam squeezing out from a doughnut when it's squashed. Either of these can occur (though prolapses are less common than once thought) and, in so doing, put pressure on the nerves in the lumbar spine.

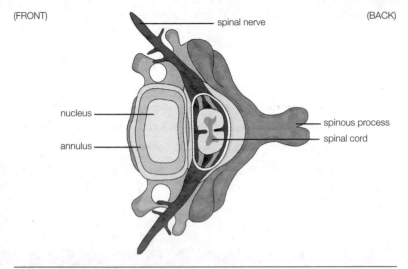

(FRONT)   spinal nerve   (BACK)

nucleus

annulus

spinous process

spinal cord

Figure 5 – Looking at a Vertebra from the top

Disc problems are less likely higher up in the spine, due to their structure and the decreased load. It is possible to have a disc bulge, or even rupture, and have little or no symptoms. It depends on whether the nerves are affected. By no means is all low back pain caused by discs. Facet strains can cause a lot of swelling and this inflammation can compromise the nerves. There are no empty spaces in your body so, if a tissue is strained and swells up, then, just like a swollen ankle, that pressure has to go somewhere and it will press on surrounding structures including the nerves. These facet strains can occur at any level in your spine and can also occur where the ribs articulate with the spine, for example, or in your pelvis.

As you'll read elsewhere in this book, there are a great many mechanisms for the production of the symptoms that people experience. Your nervous system, though, is involved in every case where there's an awareness of pain, discomfort, weakness, tingling etc. But what about those cases where there are no obviously attributable symptoms or the effects are of a more generalised nature, e.g. digestive disorders, hormonal problems or other issues? Well, the same criteria apply. These nerves can be affected in just the same way and this can lead to scores of differing conditions which chiropractic may indeed be able to help if nerve compromise is a component.

So far, we've dwelt on your spine because of it's critical role in the smooth functioning of your nervous system, and therefore your health, but what of other parts? A brief mention of some other supporting structures should be made here too. What elements of your anatomy can be involved and, briefly, how can they be explained?

Let's start at the bottom – no no, by that I mean your feet and ankles! They're composed of over 20 bones arranged in three arches, one lengthways and two crossways, to enable the foot to better withstand the forces generated in walking, running and so on. Problems can develop in these joints, which will have a profound impact on your posture and your spine. Up from there, are your knees. This is more of a straightforward hinge joint, although it does have a small degree of rotation in it, and these too can be strained and have an effect on your body as a whole. Chiropractors are trained to examine and adjust your extremities such as your feet, knees, shoulders and elbows as well, where necessary, to assist you in your recovery.

The aim here was to give you an overview of the anatomy of your nervous system and your spine in particular, given its importance in chiropractic. I hope that the small amount we have covered, will contribute to your understanding of how chiropractic can have such an amazing effect on your body as a whole, by allowing your nervous system to function at its best.

CHAPTER 6

"The greatest wealth is health."

Virgil

Prevention or Cure

By Alan Scott

We all know that prevention is better than cure but what does that mean to you? How can you prevent common health problems? Let's have a look at various aspects of preventative health and what can be done to prevent some of the most common illnesses.

Preventative health is a huge subject encompassing all aspects of our life. The prevention of disease covers a diverse set of activities ranging from washing your hands to stop the spread of germs and taking tablets to stop catching malaria when you go on holiday, to giving up smoking to prevent getting cancer and taking regular exercise to prevent heart disease.

I am sure you would like to be healthy and stay healthy forever, but what do you need to do to make this happen?

There is a growing appreciation that we need to take responsibility for our health and that our health is directly related to the choices we make. Much is made of the genetic inevitability of many diseases but we know that our environment and actions have a huge impact on our health potential (epigenetics).

The main preventable diseases are also the ones that can devastate our lives and cost our health system and society dearly. For this reason preventative health is now high on the agenda of all health policies. One of the biggest problems in preventative health is the current state of the health system itself. Most so-called health systems are actually sickness systems in that you only enter into them when you are ill, often past the point where simple measures will return your health. Thankfully, most chiropractors are well versed in dealing with preventative health issues and will encourage you in reaching your health goals.

When we look at prevention it's important to decide what we are trying to prevent. According to *The Lancet* medical journal, the leading causes of preventable deaths in the world[1] are:

Cause	Number of Deaths (millions per year)
Hypertension (raised blood pressure)	7.8
Smoking tobacco	5.0
High cholesterol	3.9
Malnutrition	3.8
Sexually transmitted diseases	3.0
Poor diet	2.8
Overweight and obesity	2.5
Physical inactivity	2.0
Alcohol	1.9
Indoor air pollution from solid fuels	1.8
Unsafe water and poor sanitation	1.6

When you look at the list, most of the items will not be a surprise and the solutions dealing with them may seem obvious. However, they continue to devastate lives and families.

The main chronic diseases that affect the developed world are heart disease, cancer, diabetes and arthritis, but rather than focusing on disease I want to focus on what we need to do to avoid these problems. The most important factor in preventing ill health is education. We all know that in order to prevent tooth decay we must brush our teeth regularly; this has been drilled into us from an early age. Unfortunately, the activities that could promote a healthy lifestyle and minimise illness do not get the same attention.

Smoking

One of the leading causes of death and disease is smoking. It is linked to cancer, heart disease and breathing problems, high blood pressure and even low back pain. I know that for some people giving up smoking can be very difficult and for others as simple as telling themselves that was the last cigarette. Have you ever wondered why we are actually able to inhale hot smoke into our lungs and not feel it? Like many of our organs our lungs have very few pain nerves; if you could feel the burning smoke entering your lungs I doubt many people would ever have a second puff.

How does smoking damage your health? The heat from burning the tobacco breaks it down and releases various toxins. Cigarettes contain more than 4000 chemical compounds and at least 400 toxic substances. As the cigarette burns, the toxins are concentrated towards the butt.

There are three major dangerous chemicals in tobacco smoke:

- tar, a carcinogen (substance that causes cancer) that forms a sticky substance in your lungs

- nicotine, which is addictive and acts mainly on your nervous and cardiovascular systems

- carbon monoxide, which reduces the amount of oxygen in the body.

The damage caused by smoking is influenced by:

- the number of cigarettes smoked
- whether the cigarette has a filter
- the way the tobacco has been prepared.

The average smoker is 14 times more likely to die from cancer of the lung, throat or mouth, four times more likely to die from cancer of the oesophagus, and twice as likely to die from heart attack.

So you can see that in many illnesses, not smoking is the best prevention.

The best option is to never have started smoking, but it's never too late to give up. There are many ways to get help with giving up smoking. It may be best to start with your government's "stop smoking" website.

Diet

The next important factor in keeping our health is diet. We all know about the dangers of either eating too much of the wrong things or too little of the right ones. Having a well balanced diet is central to health and preventing illness. Some of the major illnesses that are diet linked are obesity, diabetes, heart disease, certain cancers, high blood pressure and, of course, diseases of deficiency like thyroid problems, rickets and osteoporosis.

There are hundreds if not thousands of books out there about diet and the range of information can be confusing. One book I would strongly recommend that clarifies this issue of diet and lifestyle is Cyndi O'Meara's *Changing Habits Changing Lives*.

And a favourite piece of information I love to share when looking at making changes to diet is simple yet profound: "If you don't buy it you won't eat it."

So if you don't put it in your shopping trolley it won't make its way into your mouth.

Some simple dietary advice to follow:

Reduce your sugar intake – Sugar is hidden in many foods and may be related to many health issues but most notably obesity and diabetes, two of the greatest health challenges we currently face. However, I would warn against replacing sugar with artificial sweeteners; these are unnatural substances that your body cannot process properly.

Increase your vegetable intake (not potatoes) – Aim for more than the recommended five a day, especially dark green leafy and red or orange ones. Try and have the vegetable part of the meal first. This will fill you with fibre and nutrition and stop you eating too much of the bad stuff. Where possible have your vegetables raw or lightly steamed to keep the healthy ingredients from being altered by the cooking process.

Eat your fruit – Fruit is also an important part of a healthy balanced diet but be careful, fruit is also full of sugar. Did you know that some apples have deliberately been bred to be sweeter? Fruit is important, especially darker coloured fruit and berries as they contain important vitamins and nutrients. Juicing can also be a good way of getting your fruit and vegetables. When buying your fruit and vegetables think about eating a rainbow of colours to get as many different nutrients as possible.

Increase your water consumption – Tea and coffee do not count as they tend to dehydrate you. I would recommend at least one glass of water for every cup of tea or coffee. Your body's need for water can vary significantly depending on activity and environment. As always listen to the signals your body gives. It is very sensitive to dehydration and you will feel thirsty with only a few per cent water loss.

Alcohol

It's said that a little alcohol may actually do some good, however too much is definitely bad for us. Drinking too much is associated with heart disease, obesity, liver damage and certain cancers, and deaths related to alcohol consumption are on the increase. Alcohol is full of empty calories that have no nutritional value and simply add to your daily calorie count. Giving up the drink can be as difficult as giving up smoking so if you feel you have a problem with drink a good idea is to join an organisation that can help, or consult your doctor.

Exercise

Exercise is a key ingredient of healthy living and is known to have many preventative benefits. In fact, exercise can have a dramatic effect on health, even down to the level of your genes. Some of the health benefits are: reducing the risk of Alzheimer's, lowering levels of stress hormones, decreasing depression, helping to manage diabetes and, of course, it's an important part of weight loss.

Given how many benefits there are to exercise, it's amazing how many people don't do any at all. So what does it take to get some exercise? One thing that puts many people off the idea of exercise is the thought of having to join a gym or spend hours doing something they don't enjoy. When I give exercise advice to my patients I try and encourage them to start with simple activities and not spend too long doing them, no more than five to ten minutes initially working up to about half an hour (ideally) every day, or at least every other day.

It is thought that our ancestors walked at least ten miles per day in the course of foraging for food, so just going for a walk might be a good place to start. I also often advise using an exercise bike or cross trainer, starting gently and working up, increasing slowly each week.

When looking at what kind of exercise to do it is always best to consult a professional for advice. I explain to my patients that there are two main aspects we need to look at: one is activity that we commonly consider to be exercise, like walking, running and weights; the other aspect is stretching. Quite often the problems that we see are due to or have resulted in imbalances in muscle tone and ligament damage. Stretching is an important part of any exercise routine, but please make sure you are following good advice before you start.

Medications

Where possible avoid or reduce your medication intake. By their nature, all drugs have an effect on and must be processed by your body, which puts extra demands on your kidneys and liver. If you follow the advice in this chapter you should naturally be able to reduce some of your medication. I have had many patients tell me they have managed to stop or reduce their medications as a result of getting healthier with chiropractic care. If you are taking prescription medicine you will need to get expert advice before making any changes to your medication.

When chiropractors look at causes of ill health they often break them down into three categories: Physical stresses, Chemical stresses and Emotional stresses. This is referred to as the three dimensions of stress. So far we have covered topics that fit in to the Chemical and Physical categories; the last and equally important aspect of keeping healthy and preventing disease is Emotional health.

It is thought that one in four of us will suffer from some type of mental health issue.[2] Many people are on antidepressant medication and this does not only affect adults; children can also be prone to depression and some are even put on medication for behavioural issues.

It makes sense that if we are suffering emotionally it will affect our overall health, and the opposite is also true – poor health can affect us emotionally, starting a spiral of declining health. Often you can just tell by someone's posture and body language if they are happy or sad.

So, some simple advice to help you deal with emotional stresses. Firstly, follow the advice already given in this chapter and indeed the whole book. Then, learn to look after yourself – eat well, exercise, and stop the bad things; take time for yourself, learn to relax for a few minutes each day in peace and quiet – maybe take up a relaxing hobby. Very importantly get plenty of sleep so you are refreshed and ready for a new day. Spend time interacting with people and share your concerns; don't bottle them up. Lastly, you may want to look into EFT (Emotional Freedom Technique), which is a process of gently tapping on points on your body that can help relieve built-up stress.

In this chapter we have only touched on some of the many topics that can help you prevent ill health. Some may be easy for you to implement and get immediate benefits from; with others you may need more help and guidance. There are whole books devoted to each of the subjects I have presented and I would encourage you to become informed.

Take action now to prevent ill health in the future.

CHAPTER 7

"Changes in our lives are not new beginnings or endings, but simply the start of a new chapter in our life book."

Judith Kurz

How I Found Health

By Anna Kurz Rogers

In my mid-teenage years, back in the early eighties, I was an avid windsurfer, wearing a waist harness and sailing in the strongest winds possible. I "hurt" my back, strained it, so-to-speak, so my mother took me off to a chiropractor to have it "fixed". It was a very unpleasant experience, having to undress and pop on a gown then a man putting his hands over my back and "cracking" it!! Hence, I never returned.

That was until I was in my late 20s. By this stage I had one child, my first born son who was two at the time. I was very fit and into sports and had led my life up until then believing that going to the doctor to get antibiotics and taking Panadol, for not only myself but also my son, was the normal thing to do. My son had many antibiotics, medications etc. in his first few years and still constantly suffered from ear infections, colds, chest infections and again and again I put him on antibiotics believing I was helping.

I remember I strained my back during this period and thought it best that I find a sports chiropractor to "fix" it. This was in the early nineties. I located a chiropractor by the name of Howard O'Meara and I have never looked back – my understanding of physical health changed forever after my first experience with Howie.

In my nearly twenty years now of living my life through the wellbeing of chiropractic, this is what I've learnt:

> *Chiropractic is not about fixing a bad sore back. Chiropractic is about living well and servicing my body to function at its full potential, just as you would regularly service your car to keep it running soundly.*

Along the way I had to learn to "trust" – trust that my body could heal itself. My kids and I overcome illness by keeping our bodies well tuned via chiropractic.

An example in the early days was when my second-born, my daughter, was suffering from a high temperature. Before I understood chiropractic I would reach for children's Panadol to bring the temperature down, but through the support of my chiropractor and his wife, I allowed my daughter's body to weave its magic rather than interfering with chemicals. It was very, very difficult seeing my daughter's temperature rise and rise and I found myself picking up the telephone to ring Howard and Cyndi to confirm that what I was doing was right. They kept saying, "trust and wait". Sure enough, by the next morning my daughter's temperature had dropped back to normal and she was over her cold within 24 hours.

You see, what I learnt was that the body's temperature will rise as our immune system fights its hardest to kill off the germ invading us. It's like when we exercise, our body is pushed so our heart beat rises, breathing becomes rapid and we feel exerted. The body temperature is the same thing. The body is working hard, so our temperature has to rise accordingly. When we intervene with chemicals such as Panadol, our body or immune system is unable to work as hard to kill off the germ, thereby taking much longer to recover. It is so simple, such basic logic – how on earth can our population have missed this?

From then on, my children never had antibiotics, Panadol or any other chemical substance. My eldest son is now 21, my daughter 18, second son 12 and youngest son four.

I have learnt to trust and understand that with a chiropractic correction of the nervous system, our bodies will overcome that common cold, flu or chest infection.

I have learnt that if my body pains somewhere, whether that be my foot, shoulders, mid-thoracic area, my arm, head or even the slightest twinge in my waist area, it is working hard – I've done something wrong such as eat too much fatty food or not drink enough water, have too much dairy or not enough protein. The signs are there if you simply take the time to listen to your body. By listening, you can correct by eliminating that food or drinking more water and, of course, without question, have a tune-up – go see your chiropractor for a very quick and simple adjustment.

I've learnt that external influences, i.e. food, chemicals etc. and also emotions, are key causes of our body having to work harder to function, and consequently showing us pain somewhere. With a chiropractic correction, our body can overcome the irregularity caused by these influences with much more ease and return to its correct functioning order within a very short time.

Emotions such as stress, anxiety and grief can cause our bodies to over-function. I still, to this day, am blown away by how a chiropractic adjustment can return my scattered brain to clarity.

An example is when I become highly stressed and overtired. I have learnt that my body functions using high levels of adrenals. The stressed adrenals will cause me pain somewhere, usually in my shoulder blade and my shoulder then begins to ache so badly. I become aware, have a correction, and within 24 hours the ache in my shoulder has gone away and I begin to function at a much calmer level.

When my youngest son becomes ratty, doesn't sleep well, is overtired and naughty, I know it's time for an adjustment. A correction of the nervous system instantly calms him down and he sleeps soundly. I have followed this procedure with all my children from when the eldest was a toddler and it has worked every time. These days, if my children are not feeling 100 per cent they say, "Mum can you take me to see Dr Howard?" They don't have to be suffering from a cold etc. but they simply have learnt through their own experiences with chiropractic how much better their bodies feel after an adjustment. They have learnt that by keeping their external influences on-track via good food and water and regular adjustments, they will keep their body in tip-top shape.

My eldest children who are now young adults never follow the "norm" and take Panadol for their headaches; instead they understand that a headache is often caused through external interference, like too much sugary food. So instead of taking something for the pain they will eat only fruit and drink lots of water until their headache subsides.

There is another side of chiropractic that I have learnt and it's a procedure called NET, Neuro Emotional Technique. It simply unblocks any emotional issues being held in our nervous system and causing interference to any one of our body's organs. Again, as I mentioned earlier, I may have an ache in my lower back, just above my waist, that would indicate to me that my kidney is suffering so I must drink more water. I have learnt that if the pain doesn't go away after drinking sufficient water then maybe there is an emotional influence. Having a NET session will unblock that emotion that I may be subconsciously carrying and, sure enough, the pain goes. A NET session is not a consultation with a psychiatrist but a session with a caring chiropractor who uses simple techniques to question the nervous system by using the arm muscle as a feedback mechanism to find out what has triggered that particular emotion, then clearing the blockage.

An example of this is when I was struggling to fall pregnant after my third child. My life was consumed with falling pregnant. I did conceive twice but miscarried – the grief was horrendous and I was becoming run down and miserable, with colds taking effect on my body. I knew it was time for a NET session. As each individual organ in our body holds a certain emotion, my chiropractor questioned my body using my arm to test each organ. By determining which organ is suffering you can determine the emotion. In this case, my lungs tested positive – and the emotion was grief. It became clear to me that the reason I was getting run down and full of colds was that the feeling of grief was taking its toll on my lungs making them susceptible to the cold virus. My chiropractor then asked my body to remember a time when I last felt this pain – our *conscious* mind will not answer but, would you believe it, our *subconscious* mind listens every time and brings to the conscious mind a memory or thought relevant to that emotion. It is absolutely extraordinary! The chiropractor will then work to unblock that memory or thought of its emotional baggage, that is the blockage in our nervous system. It is over in minutes and within 24 hours you will be getting on with your day and all of a sudden it will dawn on you that you are no longer feeling that pain somewhere in your body or emotions and your head is clear of clutter. To this day, it still astounds me how our bodies are so powerful.

I live on a farm with my husband and children. I love to work hard and I adore being physical in the garden, out in the paddocks, or riding my horses. I look after the family, our animals, our business and our home. My life is busy and full and sometimes I can push my body to the extreme without really noticing it too much. But then, all of a sudden, I might bend over a certain way or move my body to pick something up or do something as simple as turning my head to look at something and, bang, my body shows me a sign. This could be anything from pain in my lower back to a locked ankle or a very stiff and sore neck. "Damn," I say to myself. "Damn! I have worked too hard and my body is telling me so." I have my corrective adjustment and my body reacts by feeling lazy and weak, but I now understand that it is simply telling me that I must not work hard for the next few days. I need to take it easy and keep my body free from any dis- ease. Again, this is such simple logic that I never understand how our population cannot see this clarity.

I've learnt that if we don't introduce chiropractic into our lives until our later years that chiropractic is not a quick fix. We must allow time for our bodies to peel back the layers of intense abuse from the time we were born. You think about it. At our births we are pushed through a very small area, twisted and often pulled out – the force on our young bodies is severe. Then comes food, often of the processed and tinned kind, and injections of the chemical kind. We then go on to learning to walk, taking many tumbles on the way, and we learn to ride our first bike and also discover that sugary food, lollies, ice-cream and cordial are so yummy. Then we hit our teenage years with high hormonal changes, lots more sugary food, chocolate and, of course, we reach the age of drinking alcohol, smoking, and the pill. And usually by this time the greater percentage of the population has suffered the loss of a loved one, a divorce and … get my drift? There are layers and layers of external influences from the time we are born that our bodies compensate for in different ways over the years. Some children become hyperactive, some teenagers go off the rails, some develop glandular fever and some adults just simply can't get their life together, feeling like they are spinning in a spiral, and often turn to drugs and alcohol.

Layers upon layers must carefully be peeled back until, bingo, health is really showing in everything we do and every way we think. Truly amazing.

However, the lucky ones like my children who have been under chiropractic care all their lives, experience very quick recoveries as there are no layers to peel back but the one that is being adjusted for. The results, for example, in my children who have gone through sleeplessness or rattiness have been instant. Another example is if one of my children develops a simple cold with a snotty nose – this tells me they have eaten too much sugary food, not had enough water and need an adjustment. I can honestly tell you that within 24 hours of an adjustment and feeding them lots of fruit and plenty of water, they are no longer suffering from cold symptoms.

My eldest son has grown up and moved out of home now, in fact to another state, but I am proud to say that he knows and understands how chiropractic works and that he, as his own adult person, takes himself off for an adjustment regularly. I expect his sister and brothers will do the same.

CHAPTER 8

"We all have choices to make in our lives – some have been better than others – but we do have a choice with how we respond to them."

Oprah Winfrey

Why I Love What I Do!

By Linda Power

When I was a child of three or four years of age, I had two recurring nightmares. One was simply about being chased by a person in a white coat with a hypodermic needle! The other was more profound. I was living with my family, friends and neighbours on a series of interlaced "Indiana Jones" bridges – suspended about eight metres above a gymnasium floor. While I was happy living there with my loved ones, I knew that over a period of time the wood would rot, the rope would rot, and I would watch helplessly as the people I loved fell through to the floor below. But that was not the scariest part for me! The part that made me wake in a cold terror was watching people dressed in white coats on that floor pick up my loved one, lay that person on an operating table, then pick up a knife to cut into that body.

They say we do what we do either out of love, hate or fear. I was so very lucky to be born into a loving family that paid close attention to health. Therefore, at age three, I had no direct conscious experience of the medical profession and I have no idea at all where these nightmares came from, but they certainly helped form my future.

My father was a forward-thinking farmer who considered himself a steward of the land and was given public honours for it. He was a pioneer in the trend toward "organic farming" before the term was part of our language. He paid attention to contour farming and crop rotation and used organic fertiliser off the farm floor. We had chickens, cattle, pigs, and sheep whose droppings he recycled to grow better crops. My mother had been a school teacher when she met him and she carried their philosophy into the kitchen. "You are what you eat" was drummed into us and we had a large vegetable garden, numerous fruit trees, and our own source of superb meat. In the autumn we would can, bottle or freeze large quantities of fruits and vegetables. We butchered our own free-range roosters and froze them. With only a three- to five-month growing season in Iowa, we had to "make hay while the sun shines" and prepare for up to six months of snow. It was a *great* way to grow up. I learned to look after the land and the land looked after me.

Maybe part of this was because at age fourteen my father fell off a horse-drawn wagon. The wagonload of kids couldn't stop and the large wooden wheel ran over his mid-section. He was hurt so badly that after months of illness, the medical people gave up on him, so my grandparents decided to take him to a chiropractor. Doctor Humphreys was practising in Atlantic, Iowa and while it was quite a trek to get Dad from the farm to the chiropractor's office, it paid off. Dad not only got better but went back to school and got his high school diploma in 1936. Then, at age 28, he fell madly in love with and married Mom. She was quickly introduced to chiropractic health care and started getting monthly health check-ups from Doc Petersen who graduated from Palmer College of Chiropractic in 1912. A few years later, my older sister was born and by the time I was born, my whole family had already had years of natural health care.

Years later I would find out that there is a Swiss genetic scientist who did a research paper on what he termed "The Predicament of the Species". He tested several families over three generations and found that humanity is degenerating genetically! Scary stuff!!! But a chiropractor asked him to repeat his study, this time using families where all three generations received chiropractic care prior to giving birth to the next generation. And this gave us hope, for in those families the genetic code was improving with each generation. Cyndi O'Meara's family is a great example of three generations of chiropractic care producing conscious, intelligent, and healthy individuals! I like to think my family has done the same.

But back to my choices early in life. School was easy for me intellectually but not so much socially. I was happier running around the fields than interacting with the cliquey groups in school. So the grades were good but I was very shy and introverted. My favourite teacher was the biology teacher who let us experiment to our heart's content, rarely gave us exams, and had me falling even more in love with the sciences. In year 11 we were given an "aptitude test" to determine what we might excel at after graduation. But when my high school counsellor suggested, based on the aptitude exam, that I study medicine, specifically surgery, you can imagine my horror! Memories of my early nightmares came flooding forward and I said, "While I may have the aptitude, I do *not* have the attitude!" He was very disappointed – maybe because I was dating his son at the time?

Next I was offered a scholarship to a teaching college, but I didn't want to be a teacher either. I didn't know what I wanted so as soon as I finished high school (actually the morning after!) I moved to the beach in California. San Diego had much warmer weather, lots of sailors, and freedom for me to find myself. But San Diego is also known as "sinus valley" so one of the first things I did was find a chiropractor for regular check-ups so that I didn't need to rely on drugs for clear sinuses. His name was Harrison B. Zook and he was a gentle, grandfatherly type of man.

I had been pondering my future for about 15 months when Dr Zook asked me what I was planning to do. When I replied that I had no idea, he suggested chiropractic. It was like a light came on! It was the sciences. It was natural health. It was conservation of the body. It was a way for me to repair and keep up the safety of those "interlaced Indiana Jones bridges"! It combined everything I loved with solutions for the things I feared and hated most.

A career in chiropractic was the solution! In college I married my biochemistry professor, the most handsome, intelligent single man on campus, an Australian student who was working his way through his studies by making use of his teaching degree as well as a degree in biochemistry. Even before my graduation, we were blessed with our own little bundle of DNA in the form of Gavin. About three and a half years later, Melissa joined our family, and they were as different as chalk and cheese. Gavin came into this world with a 37(and a half)-hour labour in Iowa City Hospital. He was practically born teething so breast feeding was extremely challenging. And he hated teething and made certain we shared his misery for about two weeks for each and every tooth. Melissa, on the other hand, was born in only two hours and fifteen minutes and landed in our hands at the side of the road, halfway to the birthing centre in Brisbane. She was a great sleeper and got no teeth till she was about ten months of age. We thought we were going to have a gummer for life, but then one night instead of sleeping through, she woke up, called out for a drink of water, and then went straight back to sleep. The next morning there was a tooth in her mouth. This little ritual was repeated with each tooth. Her teething was as painless as Gavin's was difficult. And while Gavin's first year of life was emphasised by his aggressive adaptation to planet earth – in other words, he went through the "catching bugs and fighting them off", and he did so very effectively and efficiently. His immune system was exercised and developed nicely.

Melissa had no such first twelve months. Maybe this was because she was not born in hospital. Maybe it was because she had a much easier birth. Her immune system had no real challenge for her first year on this planet, so when the baby-sitter's cat mauled her just shy of one year old, she was not ready for the viral onslaught of cat bite fever. She had been just starting to ween herself off the breast, but her best source of fluid and nutrition was my milk. So I sat in a rocking chair for nearly three months – coaxing her to drink a bit in spite of her "razor blade" throat. We had a family friend medical doctor who came around nearly daily to check on her. He advised us not to take her to hospital where she would be exposed to far too many other infections. He also agreed that, at that time, there was nothing medicine could do for a virus, so we persevered without chemical intervention. But at two and a half months into this episode, I was so distraught by her suffering that I said a prayer to God to take her if he wanted her. Because I loved her so very much, I just didn't want her to suffer anymore. And God answered my prayer, for from that point on, she got better and better. At 12 months old, she had weighed 15 pounds – a beautiful, fined-boned, rosy-cheeked baby; but at 15 months, she weighed just 12 pounds. Her immune system had suffered excessive exercise but came through. To this day, she has huge – and I mean HUGE – tonsils! So much so that when she was at boarding school, if she wanted a break, she just went to the school nurse and showed her throat. I knew that was how her tonsils always looked, Melissa also knew that, but the school nurse didn't and always gave her bed rest. Her body's immune system had done so much work at age one that her tonsils developed like a body builder's muscles. She's now 31 years old and still has those big beautiful tonsils. They've never given her any grief and have only supported a very healthy immune system – due to that unfortunate episode with the cat.

With my love of science, it's always fascinated me that a sperm and an egg can come together and then, in only 265 days, form a perfect little human being with billions of cells, all laid down in the right position. How the DNA from two cells can combine and multiply that many times without the help of modern day medicine is truly a miracle. Actually, the more interference the medical profession supplies, the more they must supply – for almost every medical treatment has side effects. I'm not saying we don't need medicine – we most certainly do, but not nearly as much as is often given. If we would just follow a few simple guidelines, we could have much more quality and quantity of life. I noticed in the July 2008 HCF newsletter (Australia) that even the medical fraternity are saying this!

1) **Have an attitude of gratitude.** I live by "As a man thinketh in his heart, so is he!" If I am grateful for each moment I am here, I will see more opportunities for health, wealth, and happiness. If I'm grateful for the fever I have, I allow the fever to do its job more effectively.

2) **Drink water.** Human beings are mostly water – males being about 75% and females up to 85%. Both male and female discs (the pads between the vertebrae of our spine that allow us movement) are 80% water. So, drink a minimum of one and a half to two litres of good clean water per day.

3) **Avoid refined foods.** White flour, white rice, and sugar – I long ago heard about a study that showed a twelve-year-old boy's immune system drops by 60 percent after one Mars bar! Sugar is hidden in abundance in almost everything from bread to tomato sauce. (See *Sugar Blues* by William Dufty.)

4) **Avoid artificial flavours, colours, sweeteners, and preservatives.** Be a label reader. When Gavin was small I learned the hard way that giving in to him about foods that had artificial flavours, colours, and preservatives did not pay. My angel would turn into a monster! Mind you, he would have the same reaction if I let him watch television for more that 45 minutes at a time. There's a book called *The Plug-in Drug* by Marie Winn with further explanation of this phenomenon.

5) **Think tall.** The primary respiration for our bodies is not through our lungs – we can do without breathing fresh air into our lungs for up to several minutes, but we cannot do without fluid flow through our brain

and spinal cord, "cerebral spinal fluid flow", or CSF flow. It's CSF flow that brings nutrients to our brain and takes away the waste products. The movement of CSF is dependent on the network of membranes in our skull and spine which must be a) balanced, b) at tension – not too much or too little, and c) in motion. Any upset in these membranes can also cause an upset in the blood flow to the brain.

And this brings us to – sitting with our knees crossed. Young women are even taught that this is the correct way to sit. (And high heels are a good thing?) Sitting with our knees crossed torques the pelvis which in turn torques the base of these membrane attachments, creating a torque through the spine. This diminishes CSF flow and creates what I like to refer to as the SBS, or stagnant brain syndrome. In my cynicism, I might think this is a conspiracy to keep women less intelligent, but I see many men sitting that way too!

6) **Get enough sleep and enough exercise.** Each of us needs different quantities of both sleep and exercise, and different amounts of each at different times. "Enough" will be a different amount for each of us and it will also fluctuate, so listen to your body about what is enough for you.

Chiropractic is not just a science and art – it's also a philosophy of health, and if we do these simple things we can keep up the health of those bridges and our precarious balance on them.

So why am I a chiropractor? Because it's taught me a healthy way of life, made me a better mother, and allowed me to share the gift of health with so many absolutely wonderful patients. I didn't want to become a teacher when I was in high school, but now I have the privilege of teaching my patients how to attain health, happiness, and longevity. And I LOVE it!

CHAPTER 9

"As you begin making significant life changes,
make sure some very important things –
principles, values, and faith – never change."

Art Berg

Evolving
Wellness

By Wayne Whittingham

Wellness is a relatively new term and has been loosely interpreted throughout different professions. It has gathered pace through knowledge, technology and understanding and the cumulative effect is changing people's lives as they get to know their bodies better, learn about nutrition, and realise that optimum health is a proactive process, not a maintenance schedule. Your body and the environment are constantly changing and you are constantly adapting as you experience new things.

Dr Gerald Smith has explained that it takes at least fifty years for big shifts in the way society accepts new ideas or new concepts as the new "gospel" to occur. This is largely because education establishes principles which a student must learn. These "truths" represent the efforts of the establishment-orientated thinkers; and in time, these principles become gospel and are used as yardsticks with which the student measures new information. Once entrenched, these principles become extremely difficult to change.[1]

Wellness is a concept embraced by all health professionals whose intent is to educate and assist their clients to live an optimal lifestyle. A little bit of education can go a long way –

> – *incorporating what might seem like tiny changes now, you can have a profound life-long effect on your overall health.*

So I'm going to address the role chiropractors play in the "wellness revolution", which has been described by some authors as potentially the next revolution in the way our society thinks.

In his book, *The Wellness Revolution*, economist Paul Zane Pilzer predicts that wellness will become the next trillion dollar industry. According to Pilzer, wellness is "not a fad or trend"; it's about a new and infinite need infusing itself into the way we eat, exercise, sleep, work, save, age, and almost every other aspect of our lives.[2]

The first revolution was the agricultural revolution whereby farmers started to produce specialised farms: some became dairy farmers, some sheep farmers, others specialised in crops or poultry. The next big revolution was the industrial revolution, the introduction of factories, dockyards etc. Currently we are experiencing the technological revolution, the mind-blowing capabilities of a mobile phone, for example, compared to ten years ago.

The wellness concept has been gaining momentum as technology has helped us understand the function of the human body on a new level. There are many definitions or interpretations of the wellness concept:

- The National Wellness Institute definition is "wellness is an active process of becoming aware of and making choices toward a more successful existence".[3]

- A more comprehensive definition is provided by Arizona State University: "Wellness is an active, lifelong process of becoming aware of choices and making decisions toward a more balanced and fulfilling life. Wellness involves choices about our lives and our priorities that determine our lifestyles".[4]

- The Merriam-Webster online dictionary defines wellness simply as, "the quality or state of being in good health especially as an actively sought goal".[5]

These definitions embrace a vision of wellness grounded in empowerment, choice and awareness. These wellness concepts sharply contrast with the more allopathic (mainstream medicine) approach, being fear-driven, patient-passive, episodic strategies of early detection, prevention and maintenance.

The human body is an amazing organism. To give a brief insight into what it's doing right now ... under normal circumstances, your body's 100 trillion cells are breaking down at a rate of 24 billion per day. In each cell there are between 300 and 800 power plants called mitochondria. Within each mitochondria in the liver there are approximately 5000 respiratory units, while each mitochondria in the heart contains as many as 20,000 respiratory units. The 70,000 miles of blood vessels that transport the body's fluids contain 30 trillion red blood cells. The normal, healthy individual produces 15 million red blood cells per second to replace the same number that are destroyed. That turnover represents 900 million red blood cells per hour.[6]

When you think about the monumental task going on inside you, you get to appreciate that maybe putting junk food, for example, or simple pain killers with potentially harmful side effects into your system, is no way to look after your body.

To explain where chiropractic fits into this picture, I am going to first discuss a little bit about how the body works. The numbers just mentioned when talking about the cells in your body are mind boggling, but what runs the show? How does any particular cell in your body know at any time what to do? For all the cells in your body to be able to communicate with one another, they need a master control system. This is your brain and spinal cord, the first organ to develop. From the minute of its inception it never stops working; it's on the job 24 hours a day, seven days a week. It also has to last you the rest of your life. It cannot afford to be damaged; hence it is completely encased by the solid bone of your skull, and your vertebral column – your spine! Your spine has been divided into 24 movable segments called vertebrae, giving you the ability to bend and twist and turn. It is so intricately designed that it allows movement but primarily it preserves the integrity of the nerve's roots that exit between the vertebrae. As the spinal cord descends the spinal column, nerves exit and supply all of the organs of the body.

Your brain performs one octillion functions a second – imagine that! These nerve impulses are sent up and down the spinal cord and then carried to the corresponding areas of the body. This process goes well unless there is a disturbance in the communicating system. This is where chiropractors play their role. Chiropractic pioneered the notion that patterns of nerve interference could be detected within the spinal systems. Because the bulk of the central wiring of the nervous system lies resident and connected to the spinal systems, any perpetual distortions of the spine could conceivably distort neural control. The vertebral subluxation complex represents a measurable pattern of spinal disturbance and neural interference which reflects the distraction of the person's natural ability to function at their full potential.[7]

One of the most important concerns a chiropractor has is the detection of vertebral subluxation (VS). This occurs when there is disharmony between adjacent vertebrae for whatever reason. The list of causes of VS is endless but the most common are trauma, posture/work, stress/emotional and lifestyle factors. When a subluxation occurs, a whole process comes into play.

There are five components to the Vertebral Subluxation:

1. **Joint Damage** – *Kinesiopathology* where increased pressure is placed on a joint through trauma or poor posture, resulting in reduced movement or even locking of that joint. This can sometimes be associated with a clicking or grating noise and, if left, creates degeneration i.e. arthritis.

2. **Nerve Damage** – *Neuropathology* where the nerve associated to the level at which the subluxation exists becomes either overactive through irritation or underactive through compression. This will then affect every tissue and organ supplied by this nerve.

3. **Tissue Damage** – *Histopathology* where the pressure of the subluxation causes swelling and irritation in an acute injury, or can lead to deformation of ligaments, discs and connective tissue in chronic cases – often without any pain being experienced.

4. **Muscular Damage** – *Myopathology* where the supporting muscles tighten or go into spasm as they work harder to maintain a balanced posture. This can create significant postural distortion.

5. **Health Damage** – *Pathophysiology* where the combination of the above can cause an overall deterioration in your health. As joints begin to degenerate, discs lose height and nerves become increasingly unable to convey vital information, we enter into a state of dis-ease.

Chiropractors detect VS by manual palpation and have access to other instruments designed to detect VS, such as thermal interferential and surface EMG (electromyography – testing the electrical activity of muscles).

The danger of VS is that we don't always know when they exist because they are not necessarily painful. This is because only one ninth of the nervous system is for detecting pain. Only a small portion of the nerve root that exits the vertebral column is pain sensitive, consequently nerve compression or irritation can result without causing pain.

Research has shown that merely the weight of a one penny coin can reduce nerve flow up to 60%.[8] This is why it is important to rule out the central nervous system and the spine for possible VS as a potential cause of health problems.

From a chiropractic perspective, your spine is very important to your overall health, so much like one would go to the dentist for a check up, it only makes sense to have one's spine periodically checked for VS. It is very common that if joints jam up in the spine and are left undetected (and consequently not treated), then with time these joints may seize up and potentially lead to osteoarthritis, for which there is no cure. Like anything in nature, if it is left to sit for too long it will seize up. Periodic adjustments of the spine keep it healthy and supple. Remember, symptoms are usually the last stage of a disease process.

Studies done on wellness care in the chiropractic profession:

- Blanks, Schuster and Dobson published the results of a retrospective assessment of subluxation-based chiropractic care on self-related health, wellness and quality of life. After surveying 2818 respondents in 156 practices, a strong connection was found between patients receiving chiropractic care and self-reported improvements in health, wellness and quality of life. 95% of the respondents reported that their expectations had been met, and 99% wished to continue care.[9]

- Coulter et al performed an analysis of an insurance data base, comparing patients receiving chiropractic care with non-chiropractic patients. The study consisted of senior citizens over 75 years of age. It was reported that *the persons receiving chiropractic care reported better overall health, spent fewer days in hospital and nursing homes, used fewer prescription drugs, and were more active than the non-chiropractic persons.*[10]

- Rupert, Manello, and Sandefur surveyed 311 chiropractic patients aged 65 years and older, who had received "maintenance care" for 5 years or longer. Chiropractic patients receiving maintenance care, when compared with US citizens of the same age, spent only 31% of the national average on health care services. There was a 50% reduction in medical provider visits. The health habits of patients receiving maintenance care were better overall than the general population, including decreased use of non-prescription drugs.[11]

With this growing body of evidence and the advancements of science, chiropractors are best placed to provide wellness care.

When one understands the function of the central nervous system and chiropractic care, it only makes sense to incorporate chiropractic check-ups as part of your wellness lifestyle. However good your nutrition, exercise program and lifestyle package, unless you're well adjusted and completely free of vertebral subluxation your body cannot function at its full potential.

We live our lives through our nervous system.

CHAPTER 10

"The good physician treats the disease; the great physician treats the patient who has the disease."

William Osler

Connecting your Mind and Body to Health

By John Swatland

We live in our minds and express ourselves through our bodies. Ideal health is when our mind and body are functioning at their best and when we are in alignment with life. The mind-body connection is the link between the two and it is why the body often gets better when we work on the mind, and our mind gets better when we look after our body.

If we were to use a computer analogy, then our mind would be the "software" and our brain and nerves the "hardware". We could say that the interface between our thoughts and the electrical nerve impulses and the neuro-chemicals actually *is* the mind-body connection.

Anatomy and physiology

Our mind is generally accepted to be based in our brain, and our spinal cord and nerves link the brain with the rest of our body. In the brain, messages are translated from our mind (software) into electrical and chemical impulses, which are then transported through the nervous system (hardware) to the cells of the body.

Mind-body healing techniques can provide healthy information or "programs" that can actually change the body function and structure and assist in healing and overall wellbeing.

Chiropractic adjustments to the spine help create an optimal nerve supply so there can be a clear flow of transmission for the life-giving messages to every tissue, cell and organ in the body.

Treating the whole person is important

In the past when we had a symptom in the body, the clinician would look for a solution or treat only the body, ignoring the mind, and vice versa. But now we know that mind and body cannot be treated in isolation. Science, medicine and chiropractic all now recognise that there is a clear relationship between our physical health and the state of our mind or spirit. It is now more accurate to see the mind and body as a continuum, as a connected whole, in order to help the whole person to reach their best health and full potential.

Spinal disorders can affect our psychological state, and pain can make us irritable, disturb our sleep, affect our confidence and distort our thinking. All of these and more can cause stress, anxiety and depression and lead to reduced immune function, illness and poor health.

Chiropractic is primarily a body-based approach that can generate positive flow-on effects in the minds and lives of many patients by removing interference to the nervous system, correcting spinal dysfunction, helping posture and breathing and relieving pain.

Healing the body helps the mind

Chiropractic has always recognised the importance of the mind in the cause and curing of disease. From the 1920s to the 1960s there existed a number of chiropractic psychiatric hospitals that reported some success with common mental disorders. Unfortunately, they had to close due to licensing and insurance issues.[1]

In their clinics today, having made physical adjustments to their patient's spines, many chiropractors see improvements in the functioning of the mind. For example, children with symptoms of Attention Deficit Disorders (ADD and ADHD) become calmer and can reduce or stop their Ritalin or Dexamphetamine drugs. Reports and testimonials of children getting better marks on school tests are also common.

Anecdotally, some patients have reported reduced anxiety levels following chiropractic adjustments and most patients report feeling better overall, even those who have presented with little or no pain or symptoms. I have observed in my own practice a number of patients with agoraphobia or claustrophobia who reported a lessening of their fears after chiropractic adjustments.

Some recent research on spinal care and psychology

Current evidence supports the fact that chiropractic treatment delivered primarily to the body may result in feelings of wellbeing in the minds of patients. A 2007 review of clinical trials on psychological responses to spinal manipulation concluded that: *"There was some evidence that spinal manipulation improved psychological outcomes compared with verbal interventions."*[2]

In 2008, the authors of a United Kingdom National Health Service review of evidence regarding psychological outcomes and low back pain commented on the findings: *"The study contributed clinically useful information that physical treatments, including spinal manipulation, have psychological benefits."*[3]

Some examples

One of my patients reported after her chiropractic adjustments that it was as if "fly wire had been removed" from in front of her vision; she could see and think more clearly. Like many other chiropractic patients, she felt that she had been given a new lease on life.

Another patient reported that adjustments had not only relieved her headaches, but her legs could function better and she could walk further than she had been able to for many years. She also reported that her diabetes improved and she required less insulin, probably as a result of being able to exercise more. She now walks to do her shopping, delivers it home and then turns around and goes out again for another walk! Her levels of joy, confidence and self-reliance are beyond what she thought might ever be possible.

Some chiropractic patients experience such rapid and profound relief from their existing condition, or experience a healing of something unrelated, that they feel a miracle has occurred – the healing may be physical, but the effect extends to the whole person's wellbeing, often clearing their mind and lifting their spirits. Certainly, at the very least, when a patient's pain goes away it puts them in a stronger position and frame of mind to address other issues in life and, indeed, to enjoy life more fully!

So what is the nature of this connection?

Nerve pathways and chemical messengers have been well established as major players in the mind-body connection.[4] Thoughts and stimuli in the brain lead to the release of chemicals that have effects in the body.

Conditions such as back pain and whiplash have well documented psychological factors associated with them.[5] By relieving back pain and physical stress, studies show that chiropractic patients will then have more normal brain function and body chemistry (i.e. less adrenalin and more "happy chemicals"), which enables them to lead a healthier lifestyle.[6] Without pain they can exercise more, which we know helps depression and other conditions[7], their posture becomes more upright and aligned, and their rib movement is freer and smoother. This assists with proper breathing, which we know helps anxiety, pain and other conditions.[8]

It is likely that chiropractic adjustments are removing mechanical and nerve interference and helping to restore the intricate electrical connections between the brain and the rest of the body.[9] At a physiological level, the blood supply to various parts of the brain may be improved, helping mental and emotional functions and promoting clarity of thinking and alertness, for example.

There are also healing processes that we cannot explain (yet!), such as those involving the placebo effect, psychic or energy healing, the use of "will" or intentional healing, so-called "quantum" healing, faith and prayer. We might call these phenomena an "X" factor in healing for now.

The chiropractic-patient-mind connection

Chiropractic philosophy has always maintained that the chiropractor makes the adjustment and the patient (body, mind and spirit) does the healing.

Chiropractic care is highly effective by itself on a physical level, but for that extra dimension or depth, it is a bonus for the patient when their chiropractor is open to healing on mind and spirit levels as well. If the patient is open too, then the healing relationship is magnified, along with the results.

Chiropractors can influence the mind of the patient, as all clinicians do, through their communication, education and caring touch. Patient satisfaction with chiropractic is extremely high and it is widely accepted that a healthy doctor-patient relationship is an important factor, improving clinical results and overall healing. The clinician's words, beliefs, attitudes and behavior are all important pieces in the mind-body connection puzzle. Successful chiropractors have an optimistic and positive attitude that creates an atmosphere that supports, encourages and empowers their patients on their healing path. The chiropractor is "modelling" healthy-mind behaviour – and hopefully modelling a healthy body too!

Historically, chiropractors have had such a strong belief in the power of the body to heal itself with chiropractic adjustments, that this strength of intention, or "will" of the practitioner, somehow activates and stimulates healing within some patients – we could call this the *chiropractic "X" factor!*

Some patients believe that the doctor "heals" the patient. This belief however, dis-empowers the patient. When both doctor and patient have the understanding in their mind that the patient's body is responsible for healing through its natural innate powers, then the responsibility for healing is in its correct place. The patient then can feel more empowered and a central participant in the healing process.

The chiropractor-patient connection

Pioneer of Integrative Medicine Dr Andrew Weil has stated: "*If we admit a mind/body connection and if we admit that we can accelerate healing processes or activate healing mechanisms through interventions at a mental level, then the impact of a doctor's belief system and a doctor's words on a patient become very important.*"[10] Integrative medicine is collaborative, using both medical and complementary approaches.

Dr Weil has spoken of the pessimism in medicine and "medical hexing" or "medical cursing"; for example, saying to a patient, "... there's nothing more we can do for you sir." This, in effect, directs the beliefs of the patient, influencing the outcome in a way that may not have been intended. The chiropractor is generally more optimistic, heartened by both the results he gets and by his philosophy, which is more aligned with nature and the natural order of life.

My personal experience of differing doctors' attitudes came from being an eight-year-old suffering severe migraines for six months after hitting my head in a swimming pool. My family doctor advised that I may have to "learn to live with it". Fortunately, my aunt recommended a chiropractor. His approach was positive and open and communicated "let's give it a go and see if the body can heal itself".

The chiropractic adjustments relieved my migraines immediately, and they never returned. Certainly, the chiropractor had the correct tools for the job, but his approach also allowed more space for healing. The powerful message I learned from this experience was not to place limitations on the degree of healing that the body or mind is capable.

In his book *The Brain That Changes Itself*, Norman Doidge reports that *"...positive bonds (between doctor and patient) appear to facilitate neuroplastic change ... so the patient can alter his existing intentions"*.[11] Neuroplasticity is the growing field of science that tells us that the brain is not fixed and rigid but can change and adapt both its function and structure, even into old age.

Doidge also notes that Sigmund Freud, who was originally a neurologist, believed that powerful positive transference (patient-doctor) bonds and feelings become *"... one of the many engines that promoted the cure."* Psychoanalysis is different from the chiropractic experience, but Freud is speaking of *"a certain warmth and positive sense of closeness"*[12] that often exists in the chiropractic setting and magnifies the patient's results.

Some "mind-related" symptoms may actually have physical causes

As chiropractic patients get better, they often report that other, seemingly unrelated, symptoms also improve. Symptoms such as indigestion, heart palpitations and asthma may have previously been diagnosed as being caused by anxiety or "stress" because no other physical or medical reason has been found for them.[13]

I recall one of my colleague's patients who had been taking prescribed medication for heart palpitations. His diagnosis was panic attacks. After a short period of chiropractic care, and with his doctor's consent, he was able to cease taking the medication as he was not suffering from the attacks anymore. The problem was physical in its origin, not mental or even stress related. It was not in his head, or even his heart, but due to his spinal subluxation.

So what mind-body techniques are available?

Modern mind-body medicine is a healing approach that uses the thoughts and emotions to positively influence the body.

Medical and alternative techniques include meditation, relaxation, visualisation and imagery, controlled breathing, re-birthing, biofeedback, floatation therapy and cognitive behavioural therapy. Hypnosis, spirituality and prayer can be included as well, in addition to the more traditional psychotherapy, psychological and other personal counselling (talk therapy).

Other less formal approaches can be learned with the help of a health professional or a life coach or in self-help books or at seminars. These include the use of affirmations and positive self-talk, life path work and even laughter therapy.

What can you do to maximise mind-body healing during your chiropractic experience?

If you have commenced care with a chiropractor then you are on the right track to healing your body. You can boost your results further by enrolling your brain and mind in the healing process. So where do you start and what techniques will help you most?

For simplicity and practicality we can look at techniques on two levels:

1) Your mind (which includes the conscious, sub-conscious and un-conscious minds).

2) Your life (which is, in many ways, an expression of what's in or on your mind).

1) Your mind

Generally speaking, in my chiropractic practice I find I can help most patients achieve between 70% and 80% improvement in their health with chiropractic adjustments; however, the remaining percentage points of change depend on the patient cultivating a healthier mind-state and/or choosing a healthier lifestyle. Every person is unique. Our symptoms may be similar, but our healing journeys toward an aligned life are personal.

(i) What is the mind?

Most people equate mind with their thoughts but, for ease, I will define it as our intellect and our consciousness. Thus the mind includes thought, perception, memory, emotion, will, imagination and the unconscious.

Healing work with the emotions, for example, has a powerful effect on both the mind and the body. Cell biologist, researcher and author Candice Pert considers the emotions to be the bridge between mind and body, as they traverse and connect both the physical and mental realms.[14]

In my experience, doing some kind of emotional processing where feelings are activated, such as in relationship workshops or counselling therapy, a greater level of emotional maturity and confidence in an individual can be reached. I have found this with my patients and myself, and this new state of awareness can then physically lead to better posture, improved breathing and more relaxed muscles. Chiropractic adjustments can then "hold" better and for longer and better overall health can follow.

In my practice, patients occasionally have "emotional releases" during or after a chiropractic adjustment, as if the body is letting go of some stored up emotion. Perhaps if the body is free of spine and nerve dysfunction, it is then freer to feel or release emotions and their blockages.

Some of my most profound healing experiences have been in the form of a realisation after emotional work that has led to a deeper level of understanding or compassion for others. It has been my experience that emotions can hold within them deep and healing life insights and when worked through therapeutically or felt fully, as opposed to being repressed or suppressed, can have positive effects on mind, body and spirit.

(ii) Meditation, for example

A whole chapter could be written on each mind-body technique listed above, but because I have broad experience with different forms of meditation over many years, I have chosen it as one example. Meditation has also achieved a high level of scientific acceptance due to the work of prominent medical researchers like Herbert Benson, who first defined the *relaxation response* in 1975.[15]

Meditation is the art of focusing the mind on a sound, object, movement or the breath in order to increase awareness of the present moment, for relaxation or to reduce stress, or to enhance personal and spiritual growth. It is a state of inner peace, tranquillity and clarity.

I first experienced this deep level of peace when practising a form of eastern Siddha meditation, and during floatation tank sessions in Adelaide in 1985. I re-visited this experience again after learning Transcendental Meditation (TM) while working in the United Kingdom in 1989. I still practise it today and believe it to be such a simple yet incredibly powerful technique that I regularly hold introductory meditation and breathing classes for my patients.

My personal physical experience of an immediate mind-body effect in the first few minutes of meditation is the feeling of tension in my shoulder muscles melting away. My spinal muscles also relax and my spine and posture become more and more comfortably upright as the session progresses. At the end of a session of 20 minutes or longer, I feel revitalised, refreshed, physically less tight and mentally more alert and at peace.

With regard to other positive effects in the body, Dr Carl Simonton, in his book *Getting Well Again*, reported that mental visualisation imagery (a kind of meditation) improved the success rates in cancer sufferers undergoing radiation treatment.[16]

Meditators also have a stronger immune response, decreased levels of stress-related cortisol and have reduced chronic pain.[17] Meditation also helps a variety of other conditions such as cardiovascular disease, asthma and pre-menstrual syndrome.[18]

2) Your life

As mentioned previously, the human brain is an organ that changes in response to its experience – it is "neuroplastic". Norman Doidge reported that in response to mental training or life in enriched environments, the brains of animals increased in weight by 5% and the nerve cells grew 25% more branches.[19] Respected mind-body researcher Richard Davidson has stated: *"our brains are intimately interwoven with our environment internal and external ... in ways that shape the physical structure ... even down to gene expression."*[20]

Professor of Medicine at the University of California Dean Ornish says that as we change our lifestyles and the way we think, then so do our brains and bodies change in remarkable and profound healing ways. He demonstrated 30 years ago that it's possible to reverse heart disease by eating a plant-based diet, exercising, meditating, practising yoga, and being part of a supportive group.

He has recently published how these practices can reverse coronary heart disease, prostate cancer and even ageing.[21]

Chiropractors will first attend to your spine and then, while it corrects and heals, help you toward a healthy lifestyle. As your lifestyle changes you think differently, and this will change your brain and your gene expression. Science is hinting that we really do create our reality.

Chiropractors want you to not only be pain-free but also to lead a flourishing life; to live to the fullest of your potential – that is real optimal health!

(i) **Practical life techniques**

When we focus on creating an environment that supports a 'flourishing mind' then there is less space in our lives for "unhealthy" thoughts.

By first making a choice for a healthier life, and then concentrating our focus, our intention or our "will" can be used as a tool to maximise our healing. As we put our attention on our healthy habits we then leave less time for the unhealthy habits, and they cease to become habits at all. (See Cyndi OMeara's *Changing Habits Changing Lives* for help with habits!)

Some action steps might include practical things like: finding your purpose and meaning in life and focusing on it; learning and practising better time management; allowing yourself to dream and setting goals based on those dreams; finding a healthy balance between work, family and recreational self-time. Other steps could include fostering more social contacts, group or community activities such as meditation groups, and even simple things like living in a clean and healthy environment.

(ii) **Keep flexible and open on all levels**

The important thing is to keep open and flexible in mind and body – to be open to all approaches of healing. No single approach is going to work for every person.

All aspects of your life may need to be explored to find healing. From early childhood trauma to current relationship difficulties, from rigid beliefs to emotional blocks such as fears, each person's healing needs are unique and personal. Variety, persistence, creativity and courage are all helpful qualities on this wholistic healing path, along with taking action of course and actually doing something!

As you progress on your chiropractic healing journey, your chiropractor will get to know you very well and will be ideally placed to make suggestions and provide personal advice and possible "next steps" to getting your life into alignment.

In summary

In the future we may wonder why we ever separated mind and body. All parts of us are interconnected and, as we heal in one sector, we are positively influencing all other sectors and expanding our overall potential. Our thoughts and feelings can change our bodies and changing our bodies can help our thoughts and feelings. Just knowing this fact is beneficial.

The spine protects the nervous system which is the information super-highway between the brain and the rest of the body (all hardware). If the brain needs to communicate messages (software) to target organs, then this highway must be clear of congestion, whether mental, physical or emotional.

Chiropractors remove this congestion by adjusting and aligning their patients' spines and promoting a culture of wellness. The chiropractor can get your spine into alignment while you get your life into alignment.

Chiropractic is not just a body thing; it's a life thing. If we receive regular chiropractic adjustments and practise complementary mind-body healing techniques regularly, then we are broadening and clearing the information pathway between mind and body and increasing our likelihood of living a long and healthy life. We are not a computer, after all. Mind and body are one. We are life!

CHAPTER 11

"All truth passes through three stages.
First, it is ridiculed. Second, it is violently opposed.
Third, it is accepted as being self-evident."

Arthur Schopenhauer

Nutrition and Chiropractic – Partners in Health

By Cyndi O'Meara

I had my first check up by a chiropractor the day I was born – from my father. I now have a family of chiropractors: my sister, husband and daughter, as well as many close friends. It has been my way of health care, along with good nutrition, for 50 years. I rarely visit a doctor nor do my children, unless of course we have a broken bone, need stitches for cuts, or encounter something that needs emergency attention that good healthy food and chiropractic can't help.

My dad began his professional career as a pharmacist but after six years he decided that dishing out medications to mask symptoms was not conducive to health. So, in 1956, he flew from New Zealand to the USA and attended Palmer College of Chiropractic in Iowa. Of course back in those days chiropractors were being put in jail for practising medicine without a license, but my father knew that this was the profession of the future and he wanted to be part of a revolution that looked at the body as an innate intelligence that was capable of excellent health.

Conventional health care today views the human body as inadequate, that it was made with many flaws, including insufficient Vitamin K at birth, an immune system that was not capable of working by itself, and not being able to handle the first pain experienced (first teeth). Conventional health care today believes that the body is incapable of curing itself, so when sickness or illness come along, it either takes the diseased organ out or uses drugs in order to try and stop the disease.

I was taught that the philosophy of chiropractic is that the body is perfect and as long as we give it the right resources in the way of food, water, air and sunlight, and there is no interference (subluxations, drugs, chemicals, toxins), then it is capable of wonderful energetic health.

This was the way I was brought up and the way I raised my children; that is, we are perfect, our body is amazing and we *can* be healthy.

> *I'm 50 and I've never had an antibiotic, pain killer,*
> *anti-inflammatory or any form of medication.*

My children are now adults aged 21, 19 and 17 and they, too, have never had any need for medication. I must add here that I am not against medications; what I'm against is the indiscriminate use of medications. If they are used wisely they have great power, but the more we consume the less effective they become. In the UK it has been estimated that the average person in their lifetime will consume 14,000 prescribed medications and 40,000 prescribed and over-the-counter medications. The latest research shows that Australians consume 14,600 million tablets a year as a nation. We have become indiscriminate pill poppers.

My family's health is a result of chiropractic care, healthy family relations, love, a positive attitude about life, and great food.

Growing up around chiropractors gave me a passion for health and I knew that I wanted to have something to do with health care. There were enough chiropractors in the family and my real passion was eating and food, so it was a matter of course that I finally found my vocation in being a nutritionist. But at university, while I was finishing off my Bachelor of Science (majoring in Nutrition) and preparing to start my diploma in dietetics, I realised that I didn't agree with what I was being taught. I didn't agree with low fat, margarine, no salt, counting calories, diet foods, RDAs (recommended dietary allowances) and meal replacements; it went totally against what I believed in and what I had been taught as I grew up, so I finished my degree and went and did some more study about the human body. I did every "ology" I could: histology, embryology, microbiology, pathology and neurology, as well as anatomy. And after five years of university I knew enough about the body and food that I felt confident to teach a very different nutrition than what was being taught conventionally.

I guess you could call me the opposite-day nutritionist. When everyone says don't eat salt, I say we need salt (but unrefined salt); if they say eat margarine, I say butter is better. I'd rather have milk straight from the cow than milk that has been homogenised, skimmed, trimmed, shaped, fat taken out, oil added to it, fibre added and all the other things they do to milk. When convention says count calories, I say what a waste of time. If everyone is doing low fat, I go full fat. When the majority is into no sugar and consuming one calorie, I eat the real thing.

You see, I believe that the health statistics, or rather sickness statistics, that we see in the western world are the result of most people doing the same thing and getting the same result – such as the increase in obesity, heart disease, cancer, diabetes, mental illness, autism, allergies and asthma; the list is endless. In the last 20 years, these diseases and many more have become out of control and they just seem to keep rising, despite the billions of dollars put into research to find a cure. So I figure if everyone is doing the same thing with their diet and health care and the sickness rate is increasing, then the most commonsense thing to do is the opposite.

Now that is the simple and most commonsense way of looking at it. But let me tell you that throughout the last 30 years I've read a lot of research on nutrition and health and I realise that the food that has been making us sick is the food that science has created, because science has this belief that the food from Mother Nature – such as butter, meat, chicken, fish, fruit, vegetables, nuts, seeds, eggs, dairy, legumes, herbs and spices – may not be healthy, and they believed in their megalomania that they could make food better. But this food from science and technology is what is making us sick.

Most people believe that food on the supermarket shelf is edible and are cajoled into buying certain foods as a result of clever marketing and advertising. Many foods now have health claims that are bogus but entice the shopper to buy for the good of their family. But let me tell you, while much of the food on the supermarket shelves is edible, a lot of these foods are making you sick.

If you are a conscious shopper you will be looking at the food label, and at present it is drummed into the discerning shopper that the nutritional panel that tells us about the fats, carbohydrates, protein, salt, sugar and fibre is of great importance. You see, we are so obsessed by the components of food that we forget to actually look at the ingredient list. People on a low-fat diet will be looking for little or no fat in a food product; those on the high protein diet will be looking at the protein amount; if fibre is important then fibre will be the focus of attention. Many times the fat, protein or salt content may be just right but if you look at the ingredients, all you see is a bunch of names and numbers, like hydrogenated vegetable oil, calcium caseinate, soy protein isolate, dextrose, aspartame, and so on. When you look at a label and you see a bunch of names that mean nothing to you, I want you to ask yourself, "Can I make this in my kitchen?" And if you can't, then don't touch that food as it has come from a chemical laboratory and not from the Garden of Eden.

The way to achieve wonderful health is no secret – it's actually just common sense – but we've lost our way and have been confounded by medical research and scientific discovery and bamboozled with jargon. This has lead to a community that no longer trusts the food from the Garden of Eden but chooses the food from an industrial kitchen/laboratory with labels that provide numbers, and behind the numbers are a concoction of chemicals that can cause cancer, obesity, neurological damage, hyperactivity and depression, to name but a few. It is no coincidence that since we've stopped eating from the Garden of Eden and started to eat margarine, flavours, artificial sweeteners, refined cereals, modified dairy and other man-made and manipulated foods, obesity, heart disease, cancer, diabetes, allergies, autism and mental disorders have exponentially exploded in the population.

I have never been about deprivation. I believe that meat pies, hot chips, chocolate cake, coffee and alcohol are foods and drinks to savour and not avoid. But the meat pie must be made with ethical meat and real gravy, and the pastry should only include the real ingredients of flour, butter, raw milk and sea salt, rather than bleached flour, hydrogenated vegetable oil, flavour, colour, refined salt and many other ingredients used to create a food that never goes off.

Once upon a time, foods were made with a few ingredients. These days, some simple foods can contain 90 or so ingredients, are unfit for human health and have been produced unethically. Some foods contain the byproducts of coal production (baking powder); others contain the backfired result of drug discoveries (artificial sweetener, for instance). You would be amazed at the underlying corruption that now stocks our supermarket shelves.

My aim is not to scaremonger but to educate in order to empower you to make food choices that will not only change your health and energy but perhaps save the population and the planet from self destruction. Imagine if the food choices you made affected global warming. Would you change what you ate? Well I'm here to let you know that what you eat not only affects global warming, it impacts on other areas too – economic policy, immigration corruption, animal cruelty, individual and overall world health, and drug abuse, to name just a few. And you thought eating was merely about filling your belly. It is important that you have knowledge about the food industry that will (hopefully) create change in the way you eat. You see I have an altruistic goal: to stop food companies making foods that not only affect global warming but are downright dangerous for you.

> *Much of the food in the supermarket may be edible but it's not necessarily good for you or the planet; in fact, much of the food on the supermarket shelf makes you sick.*

The information in my best selling book *Changing Habits Changing Lives* is like taking the red pill in the movie *The Matrix*. The red pill awakens you to the truth; if you don't read it then it is like taking the blue pill, where you continue to live in ignorance and the consequences of this choice can be devastating. Educate yourself so you can make healthy and wise choices about the food you eat, and have control of your health.

My 19-year-old daughter put it beautifully when she was seven. She told me that she had figured my book out: "God makes all the healthy food and everything else is junk." If you follow that rule of thumb, you cannot go wrong with the food you eat. Foods from nature have been eaten since the beginning of time, without the diseases we are now afflicted with in the western world.

"Chiropractic care and a healthy diet" has been my mantra and will continue to be for the rest of my life. I must stress here that I believe that there are four parts to health – the physical, chemical, emotional and spiritual – and by working on all four with the help of chiropractors, exercise, diet, love, purpose, life skills and resilience, we can live to our fullest potential.

CHAPTER 12

> *"All that we are is the result
> of what we have thought."*
>
> Buddha

The Nervous System – Your Software Program

By Linda Power

The nervous system is the computer that runs the body. According to *Gray's Anatomy*, it "controls and coordinates all bodily functions".

I remember when computers first came into use in the community at large and hearing that if they could build a computer that could do what our nervous system can do, it would take up all the room in a skyscraper.

According to one dictionary, it is a *"noun – The system of cells, tissues, and organs that regulates the body's responses to internal and external stimuli. In vertebrates it consists of the brain, spinal cord, nerves, ganglia, and parts of the receptor and effector organs."* What's that mean? It means that it's an organ in the body that monitors, records, makes sense of, and then takes the most appropriate action as far as your survival is concerned.

Just like a computer, our nervous system has hardware, software, power supply and a casing around it. And just like a computer, when there's a glitch, rarely is it the casing or hardware that is the problem. When we have a problem with our laptop or desktop computer, the problem is usually a software problem. We need to understand that our nervous system has an intelligence that it was born with – chiropractors call this "innate" (or inborn) intelligence. The problem we run into is that traumas – like a difficult birth process, falls, accidents, and illnesses – can interfere with our nervous system much the way computer viruses, bugs and other software problems do with your laptop. Our nervous system then starts to function differently – like the laptop slowing down or not working properly. This may look like faulty posture, difficulty fighting off a cold, or allergies, but these and many other symptoms are signs that your nervous system is not functioning as well as it could.

And when it's not a software problem, it's that something is not powered up or connected properly, as in a program has not been installed correctly, the switch is not turned on, or something is not "recognised"; like your computer cannot "find" your printer – even though you can see it right there on the desk beside the computer.

You've probably heard the story of the blonde (and yes, I *am* blonde!) who calls the computer shop after bringing her new computer home only days earlier and suddenly it's stopped working. The helpful person on the phone asks if it was working properly before and she answers yes. They ask if she's pushed all the "on buttons" and she answers yes, but nothing is happening. The screen just stays black! They ask if she's absolutely certain that the power is turned on at the wall, and she answers that she'll have to get a torch to check on that as there seems to be a blackout on their block and all the lights are off. The person on the phone suggests that maybe she should pack up the computer and bring it back into the shop as she's not bright enough to use it! And while this is only a joke, just like a computer, our brains *must* have a power supply. In our case, the power supply is a combination of blood flow and CSF flow. CSF flow is cerebral spinal fluid flow and while we can go without breathing for a few minutes, we cannot do without CSF flow! The fluid in your spinal cord and brain must be on the move at all times for your brain to work at all.

As a chiropractor, sometimes I feel that some patients act as though they are not bright enough to use their own brains. Like the patients who keep doing the same abusive thing to their bodies and then wonder why they're sick.

I had a patient who worked for the railway and travelled six hours each way once a month to see me. I knew he ate far too many cakes and sweets and loved the beer and advised him to make some changes. After a couple of years of once-a-month chiropractic care and *not* cutting down on the sugar foods, a warning sign appeared in his nervous system that said his pancreas was starting to feel the abuse of his diet – the pancreas is the organ that has to cope with the sugar we eat and when it can no longer cope, the result is diabetes. I begged him to cut down on the sugars, but he wouldn't. After three months of the same warning sign, I sent him for blood tests. The tests came back normal and at the hospital he was told to eat and drink whatever he liked. Three more months went by with the warning sign getting stronger. I sent him again for a blood test and again it came back within normal limits and this time they not only told him to eat and drink whatever he liked but also said rude things about the stupid chiropractor who was wasting their time! After three more months and the same neurological signs, I sent him back yet again for another blood test. This time the hospital is furious that some stupid chiropractor who knows nothing about health is wasting their time and money and she should not be allowed to practice. But they run another blood test – and this time it's positive for diabetes. Do I get an apology? No! They just tell my patient to take tablets, eat what he wants and when it's bad enough, he can go onto the injections.

I believe we have a responsibility to look after our bodies, so today if a patient won't listen to what their body is saying, I would rather not waste my time and theirs. And I do make this clear on the first patient interview these days.

Your nervous system's job (i.e. your own personal computer's job) is to monitor what is going on around and inside you and to take the right action to keep you alive! This means that if your body has let a virus in and the invader has started multiplying, your body must recognise the virus and expel it. It has a few tricks up its sleeve and the nervous system's job is to decide which ones are appropriate to use at the time. It may take your temperature right up so that the virus cannot multiply so quickly. (The increased temperature also stimulates white blood cell production, therefore increasing your army against the invader.) Your nervous system may also cause you to purge or eject the virus with vomiting, diarrhoea, a runny nose, skin eruptions and many other possibilities.

> *A healthy nervous system can eject a virus quickly and efficiently – as long as we don't interfere, and we support it with rest and healthy foods.*

Your nervous system also has a "memory pool", a bit like the memories that you can remember or think about. It has a physical record of the viruses that you have come in contact with and had to fight off, which is why a virus rarely causes you any problem more than once. That's the good part of the memory pool. But there's another side to it. All injuries that you've ever had are in there too and if the injury was not fully healed, but rather "compensated for", it alters the function of the nervous system so that now it takes on a new "normal" – not quite perfect but doing the best it can considering the trauma it's carrying. The greater the trauma, the less likelihood there is that your nervous system can fully recover its full capacity. This is the sort of problem that results in decreased efficiency of your nervous system, much like that nasty computer bug or virus in your laptop.

The nervous system is one of the first things to form in the unborn baby. At only a few weeks after conception, the brain and nervous system become obvious. It's amazing how two cells (an egg and a sperm) can come together and then all the cells are put together just the right way. We are talking millions of cells that are all put in exactly the right place according to what they are going to need to do. That must take some extraordinary innate/inborn intelligence – for a body to form – yet most people forget that and as soon as the baby comes out, *we* think we know better how it should work, so there are drugs and immunisations for nearly everything. I think I would trust a healthy nervous system much more than some years of research in a lab! If we support the innate intelligence and inbuilt healing ability in this baby body with the right nutrition, movement and a loving environment, and chiropractic care of course, it should grow into a healthy, happy and productive adult.

And how long are we supposed to live if we don't get hit by a Mack truck? I remember reading about planned obsolescence of the human body in one of our medical text books at university. It is said our bodies are actually created to last to about 120 years of age! This seems unbelievable, but I do think that we are supposed to live longer than most people do. And if this is so, why aren't doctors teaching their patients how to live longer and healthier. The most scary part of this currently accepted life span (three score and ten) that we have is, as soon as we embrace this idea, our bodies plan to live only to that age. We actually program our nervous system to run down and our bodies to fall apart. What I'm trying to say is that like a computer, our nervous system takes everything in – even our inner voice that chats away incessantly. So be careful what software you are feeding your personal computer!

The bottom line is your nervous system is your body's control system. It can be overwhelmed with too much stress, whether it's physical, toxic, or mental/emotional stress. Your body does not distinguish between the different types of stress, but just puts them all in the same basket. It does an absolutely amazing job considering what we load it up with. If we did the same to our laptop, it would definitely go on strike; but our personal computer handles almost everything – *unless that stress basket gets too full*.

So we have some alternatives:

1) Increase the capacity of your stress basket with a chiropractor who knows how to improve the health of your nervous system by working with its software and power supply.

2) Work with the chiropractor at minimising your own physical stress and toxic stress.

3) Feed your body the nutrients it needs and provide the rest and exercise that it can thrive on.

4) "Talk nice" to your body – it's the only one you have in this lifetime! Remember that your nervous system is doing the best it can and will do even better with your support.

CHAPTER 13

"All people smile in the same language."

Author unknown

When your Head and Jaw Work – So will your Body

By Mats Hansson

Cranial care, or brain care, as opposed to spinal care, involves the head! To better understand this far-reaching and essential treatment form, you need to understand the puppet analogue.

Picture a puppet with strings attached to arms and legs and every body part. The strings move to control the puppet. At the top they are all attached to a wooden block called a trestle, which allows the puppeteer to control the movement of the puppet. The puppet represents your body and the trestle is your cranium, your skull. It is obvious then that the shape of your body is controlled by the shape of your cranium.

The next analogue you need to visualise is the tepee tent. The strut in the middle (your spine) is affected by the tension in the canvas (your internal tissue). Because your body internally and externally is connected from top to bottom, any one issue – i.e. old injury, scarring, right/left handedness, fracture, operation, etc. – that affects the "canvas symmetry" would then pull on your strut (your spine) and result in faulty balance. The cumulative effect of life's many events will essentially pull at your system, causing increasing tension in the canvas and its central strut. The asymmetry and subsequent tension in the nervous system eventually leads to symptoms. Does it make sense? If your tepee tent is evenly pegged out and your centre strut is straight, you'll have a better functioning tent!

It is further obvious with these two analogues in mind that the bottom affects the top and the top affects the bottom – we call that an ascending problem (going up) or a descending problem (going down). However, most people have a combination of both! So, in order for your puppet to work and perform the way it was designed to, every string has to be balanced.

Your body is beautifully designed to perform, heal, regulate and maintain itself to its ever-changing environment, if it's fully balanced.

Due to, for example, birth trauma, accidents, stress (emotional/chemical), dental imbalance/intervention, posture habits and illness however, it can fail to keep its balance.

Chiropractic care, cranial and spinal, will assist your body to restore its balance and hence function. Chiropractors do not treat any one area (i.e. back pain, neck pain, arm or legs) but work to restore the global balance of the body – the tepee. Once the balance is returned, the body will heal itself as it was designed to do. Clever isn't it?

The History of Cranial Movement and Adjustment

History as far back as 1873 suggests that the bones of the skull fuse in early childhood. However, chiropractors and osteopaths in the early 20th century claimed that cranial bone movement existed beyond childhood, i.e. the joint – the suture, which joins one bone to the next in your cranium – moves and is essential for normal functioning of the nervous system and the entire body.

Thanks to modern testing equipment, the case was finally solved in the mid-1970s when it was established that there is movement of these sutures – approximately ¼ of a millimetre. Equally important there is also nerve and blood supply penetrating these sutures/joints to support the function of the cerebral spinal fluid (CSF), the protective layer of fluid that surrounds the brain and spinal cord. Against the medical society of the time, these early pioneers insisted that there was a rhythmic movement in all living human tissue. They claimed this cranial movement is essential and a direct expression of life – the innate intelligence responsible for the organisation of the millions of things that are constantly happening in the body.

The absence of this movement invites dysfunction and symptoms often linked with disease. Health is an active state – everything in the body moves – and not just the absence of disease.

Further research in these early years established a link between the cranium, on top, and the sacrum, the bone at the bottom of the spine. Whatever one end of the body is doing the other is reacting to – reciprocating (remember the puppet) in a very specific manner. Can you imagine what sitting for a living might do to this relationship! The brain and nervous system, which control everything, are suspended between these two parts (the cranium and the sacrum), hence this movement is essential for optimal functioning of our body. There is no medical approach for restoring this function if it's absent. The medical profession still does not recognise the presence of this system!

The Basic Function of the Cranium

The cranium (skull or, simply, the head) is on top of your body. It is made up of 26 bones. By now you have probably understood from reading this book, that your body is controlled by the nervous system. The brain, the spinal cord and all the nerves supplying every organ, bone and tissue in the body, is a two-way motorway. Very speedy information goes both ways, controlling, regulating and maintaining your system for life.

The cranium covers the brain and protects it from injury. The spinal column – the vertebras – protects the spinal cord.

Both cranial and diaphragmatic movement is controlled by a small body of nerve tissue that lies at the base of the brain known as the respiratory centre. This centre functions as the "master control", keeping perfect timing between cranial and diaphragmatic respiration. We breathe in with diaphragmatic respiration as the brain expands with cranial respiration, and the cranial bones move outward to accommodate; when we breathe out with diaphragmatic respiration, the brain contracts with a cranial respiration, and the bones retract. At the same time the sacrum, the bone at the bottom of the spine, moves – reciprocates, as discussed.

When one or more of these cranial bones are moving improperly, we have what is known as a cranial fault.

The most common cause of these faults is difficulty in the birth process. The skull of the newborn baby is very pliable. The use of forceps or ventuse on the soft skull during the birth experience can be traumatic and may cause cranial faults. Intrauterine constraints, i.e. faulty/compromised position inside prior to birth, is also suspected to contribute. Contraction-enhancing medication will also put extra pressure on these sensitive plates and may cause compression and/or misalignment.

Most severe cases of cranial faults develop before the age of seven; however, people develop cranial faults later in life from traumatic accidents such as car crashes or blows to the head. Emotional trauma is also a known cause of cranial faults and should not be overlooked. Severe emotional stress causes the body to adopt a defensive torque position in which the spine and skull receive as much punishments as if they had undergone physical trauma. Dental work may alter the function of the cranium. Teenage extraction and braces often distort the cranium and cause symptoms – not to mention dental cosmetic work where the aesthetics are prioritised and function is forgotten! Continuing research will discover more about cranial faults

The temporomandibular joint (TMJ), the jaw joint, is part of the cranium. It is where the lower jaw meets, articulate with the ear, the temporal bone. If you put your finger in your ear and open close your mouth you will feel the movement of the TMJ on the forward wall of the ear canal. Can you imagine what a blow to the jaw might do to the function of the ear? Or, if you had no teeth on one side, either up or down? Or if your teeth were pulled out in your early teens and strapped back with a brace restricting the movement of the cranium and altering the shape of the bite and the shape of your face? Basically, it will upset your "trestle" and produce symptoms either immediately or gradually as the trestle asymmetry affects the whole body! Dental associations across the world are increasingly recognising this effect and are now beginning to work together with chiropractors to better assist the patient in restoring health. The SOT association (sacral occipital technique) assesses this interlinked function.

Imagine the cranium is crooked, how then does the jaw joint line up? Not very well, hence there is no point treating only the TMJ. Likewise if the pelvis is crooked, which affects the alignment of the cranium and subsequently the jaw, there is no point treating only the TMJ. (That old song about the body parts all being connected makes sense.) I strongly urge you not to have any dental work done to yourself or your children without making sure that your dentist works together with an SOT chiropractor. (A good website to explore about this is www.orthotropics.com.)

Basic Function of the Nervous System

All the shaded bones/plates you see in figure 1 join together to form a continuous casing for the brain.

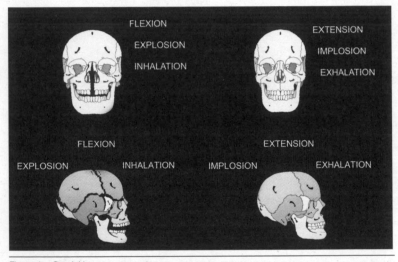

Figure 1 – Cranial bone movement

Inside or underneath these plates, the brain is suspended from its "roof" a bit like a spider in the middle of a symmetrical spider web! These web-like fibres are called meninges and they hold the brain centred in its cranial vault. Can you picture it? Yes, your third and final analogue.

From this upper centrally placed nerve centre, the brain, comes the spinal cord. The spinal cord then travels all the way down the spine until it reaches the lower spine. Here the cord ends and supplies nerves all the way down to the coccyx, the tail bone. The meninges follow the cord all the way down making sure that it stays centred in the column. So clever!

What happens do you think if you bring your chin towards your chest to look down? Does the spinal cord pull up inside the column or does it push down? Right, it pulls up! And what happens to all the nerves – the 31 pairs that exit along the way, supplying every tissue organ and bone in the body? Right again – they pull up too!

The plates of the cranium are softer at birth and gradually harden during the first six years of life. They then calcify to become hard shell to provide protection. However, in between each bone/plate the movement is maintained as discussed, which is essential for a fully functioning nervous system.

Remember the CSF – the fluid that protects, shock absorbs and nourishes the brain and maintains a very clever balance essential for the true function of the brain and hence our body, what do you think might happen when a toddler falls and bumps his or her head on the coffee table? The bone often hit is the frontal plate – the one that goes across above our eyes, commonly known as the forehead.

It will depress this bone and alter the pressure in the space below where the CSF is protecting the brain. And what function does this part of the brain provide? This area is responsible for behaviour, concentration and memory!

Hence this altered pressure affects the ability of the brain to function as designed. Remember the spider web holding the brain suspended in the centre, what happens then when one of these insertion points, i.e. the one underneath the compressed forehead bone, is no longer keeping the symmetry? It will have a knock-on effect on the tension of the brain and spinal cord and hence alter the function of the *entire* system – not just locally!

Remember the three analogues: *the puppet, the tepee tent* and now *the spider in the spider web*!

Chiropractic care restores the balance of the body, the cranium and spine to enable the full expression of health.

Symptoms of Cranial Faults

Considering the puppet analogue, symptoms of cranial faults may affect the whole body.

Babies – excessive crying, restless sleeper, poor feeder, (can't suck properly) recurrent infections, colic, projectile vomiting, head banging and/or arching back, constipation, facial, pelvis or spine asymmetry, head asymmetry (plagio cephaly) retained reflexes (see below).

Toddlers – recurrent infections, behaviour variations (autism, ADHD ADD, OCD, Asperger) head banging, speech impairment, uncoordinated (dyspraxia), slow learner (dyslexia), poor writing and/or hand control, constipation, indigestion, not thriving, bed wetting, growing pains, asthma, eczema, foot disorders, visual impairment.

Teenagers – growing pains, headaches, indigestion, constipation, inflexible, muscles pulling (sports), clicky jaw joint, failing to thrive, poor posture, fatigue, spinal and/or arm/leg pain, scoliosis, menstrual difficulties, learning difficulties (maths/reasoning, etc.), and behaviour difficulties.

Adults – pain, numbness, pins and needles, weakness, vomiting, nausea, constipation/diarrhoea, indigestion, spinal restriction, joint pains, arms/legs/ shoulders, headaches, migraines, sinusitis, waxy ears, epilepsy, jaw locking/ clicky, blood pressure, asthma, eczema, irritable bowl, loss of smell/taste.

Post concussion – headaches, blurred vision, speech difficulties, memory lapses, brain fog, emotional irregularities, decreased reflexes, altered coordination/ balance, behavioural changes, nausea, fatigue.

Retained reflex may cause – poor balance/coordination, motion sickness, sensitive to light , sensitivity to certain noises, allergies/decreased immunity, recurrent infections, adverse drug reactions, fatigues easily, dislikes change, hypoglycaemia, difficulty in making decisions, low self esteem and insecurity, cycles of hyperactivity followed by fatigue, mood swings excessive reaction to stimuli, anxiety, poor manual dexterity, unable to hold pen properly, mouth movements whilst writing, speech difficulties, unable to crawl, difficulty operating object from one hand to the other, poor handwriting and inability to express on paper, hunched posture, toe walking, apelike walk, w-leg position when sitting on floor (i.e. sitting on your knees with feet out on either side, not under your bottom), difficulty in learning to swim, poor eye hand coordination, slow to copy tasks, developmental delay, heel walking or toe walking.

TMJ dysfunction may cause – clicky or locking jaw joint, limited opening, tinnitus, decrease in hearing, ear ache without infection, increase of wax (itchy, clogged ears), vertigo/dizziness, headaches, neuralgia (pain on either side of face), Tic douloureux, Bell's palsy, sinusitis, bruxing (clenching and grinding the teeth), excessive wear of teeth, swallowing difficulties, sore throat with no infection, voice irregularities, infrequent coughing or constant throat clearing, involuntary biting of inner cheeks/lips/tongue, pelvis imbalance, low back pain, hip dysfunction, neck pain or arm pain, cranial distortion with subsequent body dysfunction (remember the puppet – i.e. crooked jaw affects the trestle).

Cranial Treatment

Cranial treatment involves pressure exerted on parts of the cranium to restore movement and balance. Depending on the age of the person and the reason behind the cranial fault, the techniques may vary. It is essential to recognise birth trauma and its effect on the cranial plates to correct these as soon as possible. We recommend that all babies should be screened by a chiropractor for any symptoms or signs relating to cranial faults. Increasingly, midwives are recommending cranial checkups following birth complications (cord around the neck, forceps/ventuse, prolonged second stage, use of contraction-enhancing medication, low apgar score, inductions, epidurals, episiotomies, emergency caesareans).

Due to the development of the cranial bones, it is more difficult to alter their shape after the second birthday. Considering the developing spider and its web, the more symmetrical the casing is, the better functioning web you get! The brain is, of course, also always developing and is sensitive to pressure changes in the surrounding CSF.

Well, I think you have the idea by now – the three analogues and their considerations on the full function of the body. Chiropractic cranial care examines for the presence of cranial faults and restores them, leaving the body and its immune system to do what it does best – keep us healthy!

CHAPTER 14

"Man who says, 'It cannot be done',
should not interrupt man who is doing it."

Chinese proverb

Immunity Boost

By Jennifer Layton

Immunity is when your body's own defences kick in to fight invading bacteria, viruses and other nasties that cause disease, along with an ability to fight cells produced by the body that are hostile, such as cancer cells. The immune system can go haywire and attack our own bodies, which can then create autoimmune disease and allergies.

Where exactly is your immune system? It's found all over the body, not just in one location; it's in the lymph, the blood, around the intestines, the bone marrow, the tonsils and the adenoids. All these areas have the benefit of a nerve supply – the nerve system controls every cell in the body. More on this later.

The development of your immune system is most significant during your childhood years. Granny was right when she let you eat the handful of dirt in the garden. Chewing on the dog's ear was not such a bad thing. When you are young, exposure to common microbes and bacteria is vital to developing the immune system. These germs might never result in clinical disease, but they do play an important part in the formation of a healthy immune system.

Your immunity is particular to yourself, and can depend on various factors. Whilst the genetic factor can't be altered, you can help your immunity to function optimally by, for instance, having excellent nutrition, doing some regular exercise, reducing the amount of toxins you are exposed to, and having some exposure to diseases. Research is also showing that chiropractic adjustments can help to improve your immune system function.

Chiropractic's connection with immunity was first noticed in the USA following the worldwide Spanish flu epidemic of 1917 to 1918, in which it has been estimated that 50 million people (or 3% of the world's population) died. It was observed that those who had been having chiropractic care fared much better than the general population. In fact, the chiropractic patients had an estimated death rate of 0.25%, and the rest of the population not receiving chiropractic had a death rate of 5%. That's a twenty times better chance of survival from the flu epidemic because of chiropractic.

So let's see what's been found with research. As stated earlier, the nerve system controls everything in the body, including the immune system. That the nerve system is involved with immunity was shown in a 1992 study, in which a mid-back adjustment (just around the shoulder blades) produced an increase in the disease-fighting white blood cells just 15 minutes later. This was significantly higher than 15 minutes before the adjustment, and 30 minutes after. This phenomenon was called an "enhanced respiratory burst". These white blood cells are like the body's pacmen, gobbling up all invaders and intruders, so you can see this is a useful effect if you are ill.

What else has shown this connection between the nerve system and immune system? A 1997 study using a chicken's spinal ligament, again from the upper back (just between its wings), showed that receptors that pick up the movement in the spine then fire off the nerves that go to the immune tissue. This shows it is so important to keep the spine moving and free from restriction or else the receptors fire incorrectly, which then compromises the body's immune system. We're not talking about the big movements of the body, but the little movements that do the stabilisation that you probably can't even feel your body doing. This is particularly relevant to posture, where these little muscles play an important role.

Off to another lab now. An investigation into the link between chiropractic and immunity compared the immune systems of those under chiropractic care, firstly to those in the general population and then, secondly, to those with cancer and other terminal illnesses. It was seen rather spectacularly that the first group of regular chiropractic patients had a 200% increase in immune function compared to the group of the general population, and a 400% increase compared to the other group with the illnesses. This is a 2 to 4 times increase in immunity that was seen – alltogether a handy effect when you consider that each day your body produces 100 to 10,000 cancer cells. These genetic mistakes randomly happen in the course of your body replacing billions of cells daily, and the immune system has to be strong to ensure these rogue cells are suitably dealt with. The immune system must be kept in top condition and not allowed to become weakened.

One more study needs mentioning. This study, in 1994, looked at a group of HIV positive patients who had their upper necks adjusted over a six month period, and compared them to those who didn't. The adjusted group had a 48% increase in the type of immune cells most affected by AIDS, yet those without the adjustments experienced an 8% decrease in these immune cells over the same period. Sadly, at this stage the funding was cut and patients not made available anymore, so no further research could be done.

Enough from the boffins, now let's look at what stress can do to the immune system and how this can relate to chiropractic.

There is plenty of literature showing that psychological stress can decrease some aspects of the immune response; that is, emotional stress can lower the strength of the immune system. We've probably all experienced getting ill when feeling stressed, usually just a cold, sometimes something worse. One of the stress responses of the body is to increase cortisol (produced by the adrenal glands, just adjacent to the kidneys). Cortisol acts to increase the blood pressure, increase blood sugar levels, and leads to a decreased immune function and an increased perception of pain. This, again, is where chiropractic steps in. By restoring nerve system function, these changes can be reversed and normal service can be resumed; that is, pain decreased and immunity restored. The chiropractic adjustment stimulates a part of the brain (the vermis, Latin for worm! It looks like a worm and is positioned in the base of the brain) which then coordinates stress reduction, increases feelings of pleasure and relaxation, and results in a decrease in susceptibility to disease and an increase in general health. It also works the other way too, where a problem with the tiny moving segment of the spine at any level can increase warning messages back up to the brain, which in turn increases the stress response. Here once more is where chiropractic can come to the rescue, restoring the movement to the segment, which in turn sends the signal back up to the brain (that's right, to the vermis again!) to shut off the stress response. Then those stress hormones go back to an appropriate level, which helps the return to a healthy immune system.

And what about the way conventional medicine might view the enhancement of immunity? It's viewed mainly from the aspect of the outside-in, not from the inside-out, as we have just been looking at. Conventional medicine would be trying to help it along by removing sources of germs and infections via cleaners and disinfectants, thereby not giving the body the important exposure to the germs that it requires. It would be treating an infection with antibiotics so the immune system doesn't then get to do this. It would be bringing a fever down by using paracetamol, a fever that is the body's way of dealing with the infection. And then perhaps surgery to remove the offending body part.

It is important to note that this is not suggesting that it is never okay to use a drug to treat a symptom. There may be a time when it is necessary to get through a crisis or an acute situation.

Further research needs to be performed to fully understand just how much
chiropractic can influence the immune system. Chiropractic should never be
described as manipulation to reduce symptoms; it is scientifically proven that
proper function of the spine is required for proper function of the nerve system
and therefore all that the nerve system reaches – which, of course, includes the
immune system.

Many chiropractic patients report suffering fewer colds, avoiding any bugs
doing the rounds, or just simply recovering from illness more quickly. Here we
have seen the scientific reasons for these observations.

CHAPTER 15

"To be pregnant is to be vitally alive, thoroughly woman, and undoubtedly inhabited."

Anne Buchanan and Debra Klingsporn

Healthy Pregnancy, Healthy Birth, Healthy Baby

By Alan Brown

The birth of a child is one of the most meaningful moments in anyone's life. Alongside the joy and wonder of conceiving a child, many people experience a sudden and almost frightening sense of responsibility. They also begin to make some serious decisions. With so much information and so many points of view available, the whole experience can be a little overwhelming.

The body of research supporting the benefits of chiropractic continues to grow and this chapter offers commonsense information about how chiropractic can help you to achieve the best pregnancy and birth possible. Whatever health care decisions you make throughout pregnancy, birth and beyond, chiropractic can be of incredible value to you and your family, giving you a more comfortable pregnancy, an easier birth, faster recovery, better breastfeeding, and a relaxed and healthy child.

You may be surprised about the range of health areas where chiropractic can lead to better outcomes; however, once you understand the principles underpinning chiropractic, the possibilities will become clear.

Many people believe the benefits of chiropractic are limited to fixing or helping spinal problems like back pain.[1] While chiropractic has achieved international recognition for its potential in this area, its scope goes far beyond the spine.

The spine houses the nervous system, the master control system that coordinates and controls the function of every system in your body. The nervous system completely controls the immune, respiratory, and circulatory systems, your thoughts, and even your posture. Vast amounts of information pulse down from the brain, along nerve pathways, and down the spinal cord to all parts of the body to maintain perfect balance and health.

Your spine is made up of 24 moveable segments (bones) called vertebrae, plus the sacrum, tail bone, pelvis and skull. Nerves branch out from the spinal cord between the spinal vertebrae. When the vertebrae are unable to move correctly, nerve interference can result. Even skull bones can move[2], and though these movements are small they are significant enough to affect our nervous system.[3]

Your health and vitality are compromised when there is any type of nerve interference or damage that interrupts normal nerve flow. Think of it like static on your telephone. A clear message is not getting through, so the body cannot coordinate its billions of activities as effectively. Chiropractors call interferences to nerve flow "subluxation". Ensuring proper communication between nerves is especially critical during pregnancy, a time when the baby is growing and developing rapidly.

Subluxations are caused by overwhelming stress – *physical, mental, emotional or chemical*. The subluxation is essentially a defence mechanism; it locks the vertebrae and surrounding tissues out of their normal position to prevent further damage, just as a fuse in your house blows when an electrical system is exposed to excessive voltage.

Subluxation is more common in pregnancy, due to the added stress of weight gain, hormonal changes and changes in sitting, standing, walking and sleeping patterns.

> *The main job of a chiropractor during pregnancy is to correct subluxations to stabilise the shifting spine, rather than to treat a particular condition.*

That said though, chiropractic care can resolve a range of symptoms including back pain, digestive problems, heartburn, headaches, sciatica, fluid retention and uncomfortable foetal position.

Let's look at some practical examples of how a subluxation can affect the pregnant mum, the birth and baby.

The sacroiliac joints, at the back of the pelvis, are highly influential, particularly during pregnancy. The sacrum can easily move out of position and become subluxated when stresses (or our sedentary lifestyle) cause the ligaments around the joint to become loose. The space between the sacroiliac joint can then widen, causing one of the larger back muscles to contract above it to support the spine against gravity. This muscle, the latissimus dorsi, attaches along the vertebrae of the mid-back and up into the ball of the shoulder joint. The continual pull of this muscle caused by the sacroiliac subluxation can result in pain in the shoulder and knock-on problems in the arm and elbow. It can even lead to carpel tunnel syndrome.

The pull of the latissimus dorsi muscle where it attaches to the mid-back (thoracic spine) can also subluxate vertebrae in that area. These thoracic vertebrae in turn influence the stomach, pancreas, and gallbladder[4], and can manifest in digestive problems such as gas, bloating, indigestion, heart burn and reflux.

Getting in and out of a chair or rolling over in bed can be difficult with an unstable pelvis. Even putting weight on one leg may cause the leg to give way from under you. I recently worked with a mother who was told by numerous health practitioners that she would have to be in a wheel chair leading up to the birth, due to these types of pelvic problems. After gently adjusting her pelvis, she regained full function within two weeks, and was more functionally capable at 38 weeks than she had been at 20 weeks.

Subluxation of the pelvis can have still more impacts. They involve other muscle groups that flex and rotate the hip (the psoas and piriformis muscles). These muscle groups become involved as the twist in the pelvis drags through the lumbar spine, causing it to rotate as well. It is amazing how often it feels like a hip problem is going on when it is actually the muscle bracing and contracting from the sacrum to the hip.

The psoas muscle runs from the ball of the hip joint, across the sacroiliac joint along the side of the lumber vertebrae and disc, and attaches into the diaphragm. Its protective contraction can even start compressing the discs in the lower back[4] and further constrict the stomach, aggravating digestion. The constricted muscles can also impact the environment around the baby, limiting its room to move. In some cases, this can cause parts of the growing skull to develop asymmetrically. The function of a baby's cranium has a huge impact on the rest of its developing spine and nervous system, a concrete example of the adage: "As the twig is bent, so is the tree."

Bear in mind that all of the effects discussed so far relate only to one subluxation occurring in the pelvis.

There is also a more sinister effect which can be caused by a pelvic subluxation.

The pelvis and sacrum are securely attached to the uterus with ligaments from behind, at the sides, and in front. If the pelvis twists out of its normal alignment then the ligaments will pull unevenly through the uterus, creating intra-uterine constraint. This can effect foetal position and development, resulting in a very difficult birth process. "Dystocia" is the name given to a lack of progression during labour, or the baby getting stuck in the birth canal. It is widely acknowledged that the diameter of a woman's pelvis is decreased when the sacrum is displaced.[5]

Here we have considered just one example of a subluxation and its possible effects on the mother, including a range of potential symptoms. When you consider this problem may not have any symptoms but could interfere with the birth process, the best advice is, don't wait to see if it starts to hurt before you get it checked. Like many other problems in the body (including diseases) you generally have the problem long before symptoms start. In fact, you may have pelvic subluxation and no back pain at all.

Chiropractic offers more than one hundred different techniques to effectively correct a subluxation like we have just discussed. These procedures are exceptionally safe. One technique, called the Webster technique, has been subject to several studies, and demonstrated a 92 per cent success rate in improving a baby's position.[6] This procedure is in no way trying to push the baby into position. The baby moves of its own accord – because it can.

The benefits of chiropractic do not end once the birth is over. It is well established that both natural and medically assisted birth processes contribute considerable stress through an infant's spine. It makes perfect sense to have your chiropractor check the infant immediately after the birth. In Denmark, most children who receive chiropractic care are babies younger than four months old.[7] This is at least partially because of a widespread understanding in the Danish community of the effect the birth process can have on an infant.

A chiropractic check-up is important for newborns because children's upper necks are especially vulnerable to subluxation. The shape of the joints in the upper neck of an infant leaves it less protected in the first months and years. The problem is further compounded by the fact that head weight relative to the body is much higher and children do not have well established muscle control between the head and trunk.[8]

In a recent medical publication, 114 infants diagnosed with breastfeeding problems in a hospital were checked by a chiropractor who found neck subluxation in 89 per cent of the infants, along with inadequate suck reflexes. As a result of chiropractic care, all children showed some improvement, with 78 per cent able to breastfeed exclusively within a 2-week time period.[9] The last thing a new mother needs is the stress of not being able to feed her baby properly, and probably blaming herself when the infant has a subluxation that goes uncorrected. These days most people are aware of the long-term benefits of breastfeeding. This is an example of a small problem having a massive long term impact on a child's health.

The infant nervous system develops rapidly after birth, with the brain growing about 400 to 1000 grams in one year. During this year, the foundations are being laid for how your child will perceive the world through each of their senses. The development of the spine and nervous system is intimately connected to the optimal function of perception. They will affect the way the eyes will lock into catching a ball, reading a book or balancing on a beam. It is important that any misalignments are corrected before pathways are laid down in a more permanent way.[8]

Beyond birth and post-natal care, subluxations in the neck are linked to ear infections in children and to the development of problem headaches – conditions which also respond well to chiropractic care.[10,11] One medical researcher described how spinal-related symptoms can manifest in the early months as anything from feeding problems to signs of colic. Then, as the child begins to walk, their nervous system develops rapidly and most symptoms seem to disappear. People sometimes believe that this means a child has 'grown out of' a particular condition; however, there are clear links between early spinal problems and disorders later in childhood or life, ranging from headaches to sensorimotor dysfunction.[8]

Chiropractic can provide benefits at so many stages of life across a broad range of symptoms; however, the greatest benefits of all lie in its promise for realising long term human potential. BJ Palmer, the developer of chiropractic, said:

> *You never know how far reaching something you think, say or do today, will affect the lives of millions tomorrow.*

This statement is particularly applicable to pregnancy and birth. There is no time of life where as much physical, chemical and spiritual change occurs. A small subluxation can be corrected before it becomes a condition that will have implications across a person's entire life.

Chiropractic can be described as the science of things natural. It works with your body to remove interferences that may occur within the nervous system and, as such, is a critical component of birthing care. However, birth can be an unpredictable process and we are fortunate to have excellent medicine available to manage birthing emergencies. Even where such situations occur, chiropractic is important to help a mother and child rebuild, recover and repair.

While the full potential of chiropractic is still being realised across our community, the evidence demonstrates its usefulness in providing the best start for its children. Chiropractic will continue to grow through its wholistic understanding of prevention, care and support through pregnancy, birth and beyond.

CHAPTER 16

"Birth is a powerful initiation, a rite of passage for all involved, which enables us to create a beautiful Life on this planet. It is our birthright!"

Elena Tonetti-Vladimirova

Trust My Body, Trust My Baby

By Kathy Knight

Growing up, my only experience of anyone having a homebirth was an aunt who, in my family's opinion, was a bit of a hippy and it was not something "normal" people did. Having grown up and become a chiropractor, however, I realised homebirth had its place, but I never really considered it as an option for myself. It was not something I particularly aspired to have or had any major belief in or thought would make any difference.

My homebirth came about because of the experience I had with my first birth. Both births are precious to me and I value them equally. I don't like to think of one as good and one as bad because one led me to the other. If I hadn't been challenged by the system and by myself physically and emotionally I would never have had the knowledge or courage to take the steps required to take charge of my second birth.

I have a strong belief in the body's ability to birth and that pregnancy and birth are normal events that do not require major medical intervention. When I found out I was pregnant with our first child I dutifully went to the doctor's, not to find out I was pregnant but to tell him I was. I'm not really sure why I went; it just seemed the thing you do when you're pregnant. Being a chiropractor and having chiropractic as my choice of health care, I hadn't been to a medical doctor in 10 years. He gave me some advice about maternity options including obstetrics, birth centre and public hospital. He mumbled something like, "I hope you're not considering a homebirth," but at the time I wasn't so I let it slide. I said I wanted as little medical intervention as possible so he steered me in the direction of the Birth Centre and the Canberra Midwifery Programme, told me to get Janet Balaskas' book on Active Birth and said to "swing from the rafters" to reduce the labour time.

I was on a steep learning curve about pregnancy and birth and the politics involved from an insider's point of view. I had provided chiropractic care for many pregnant women but was in for a big wakeup call. I realised my beliefs were well aligned with the midwifery model of care and was grateful to find it existed independently of obstetric care, which I knew instinctively to avoid. The Birth Centre seemed to be my ideal place to birth with a midwifery model of care within the hospital in case a freak emergency should arise. I didn't have to face an obstetrician and feel intimidated about my birth choices. I believed I would be able to suppress my anxiety about hospitals and medical doctors as giving birth in the Birth Centre wasn't really being in "hospital" (note: yes it is).

I was initially very happy with the Birth Centre: all my choices were respected without question; my birth plan was accepted without a batter of an eyelid; and I felt I was in good hands with a midwife who understood my wishes. I saw what I wanted to see and ignored warning signs I should have paid attention to. As I approached 42 weeks gestation however, the cracks started to show in the philosophy of care. I was pushed to have ultrasounds against my wishes and I had threatening appointments with obstetricians who tried to intimidate and scare me with ridiculous statistics about death rates of overdue babies. There was no belief in the body knowing what to do. I was completely well and healthy with not a sign of any complication that would warrant any intervention. Dates of induction started to be brought up. I was surprised because 38–42 weeks is considered full-term and since I wasn't over at this time I was confused by the advice I was receiving. Some of the midwives at the centre were able to protect me from the obstetricians wanting to interfere while others were intimidated and led me straight to the door.

Thankfully I went into labour with my first daughter at 41 weeks and six days gestation, calmly at home having dinner watching TV, and without induction. First time jitters got my husband calling our midwife who settled us and told us to call back if labour continued to progress – we had already had one false start earlier in the week. Around 9.30 pm Rob called her back and asked her to come over. By 11 pm we were heading in to the Birth Centre. I hopped in the bath, excited it was finally happening. My husband called my parents and support friend to tell them where we were. He spoke to Dad and said he would call back later as we got closer to the birth. He could only leave a message on the answering machine at my friend Michele's.

It wasn't long before I realised my birth plan was not being followed and my choices were not being respected – it was as if my plan hadn't even been read. First there were suggestions my membranes should be broken, which I'd specifically asked not to be done, yet we'd only been there for an hour. If there is one thing I can guarantee will happen on its own, it's that membranes break, although babies can be born with them still intact and if they are still intact they can cushion the birth canal. So I was starting to think there must be something wrong and tried to push the idea away. I declined the offer three times and told the midwife they'd already broken but she still called the obstetrician because she wasn't certain whether there was any membrane left and didn't want to scratch the baby's head. I felt like screaming at her to leave me and my membranes alone. The obstetrician confirmed they had already broken (thank goodness), and the second request for minimal vaginal examinations had been blown out of the water. And there was a student medical doctor observing who was talking out loud giving a running commentary on my breath control, which was rather disrespectful and distracting.

My next surprise was the suggestion to put a catheter in because I hadn't passed any urine recently. I expected a midwife would suggest I drink some more water first or, if she hasn't been observing how much I had been drinking, ask my husband who could tell her I had been drinking plenty. We also found out in hindsight it had only been an hour since I had last passed urine anyway, which isn't a long time for not peeing during a birth. I started to have images of fistulas (don't read *Hospital by the River* before having babies). I decline three times before thinking, I don't have a choice. They discover there is no urine in my bladder (which my body already knew and why I haven't peed in the last hour) so this puts me on the intervention route of requiring a cannula and IV fluids. I still couldn't understand the midwife's actions as I presumed she would encourage me to drink more before doing this, especially as I had declined the IV three times before being pressured into submission again. Where had the midwifery care gone that was so promoted as being for the woman? At this point I realised my midwife knew nothing about me or my beliefs and understanding of a birthing woman. I had expected her to own this respect more strongly than I did.

I knew all these procedures were unnecessary but I felt powerless to stop them. If I had been in the hospital or under obstetric care I would have expected them and been prepared but I had let my guard down because I was part of the Birth Centre. Every time a new procedure was brought up it was taking me away from the birthing state. I couldn't trust the midwife to look after me or that she had my best interests at hand. My anxiety levels were rising and I had no belief that the midwife was supporting me – she appeared more interested in performing procedures for the student doctor. My friend and parents hadn't arrived either. Mum and Dad were waiting for a call they were never going to receive because Rob was the only one hands on supporting me and didn't want to leave me to pick up the phone. Michele didn't get the message until 7 am. It happened I had an anterior lip which wouldn't budge. (This means I was all dilated except for a small lip at the anterior part of my cervix – which in medical terms means I can't push or I will damage my cervix or baby as it will swell. It's the reason why many births end in a caesarean.)

No wonder, with the stress I had been placed under; my body was starting to think this wasn't a safe place to birth right now and stopped dilating. There had been no respect for letting me birth as my body knew how, in the timeframe that my body and baby required.

My body started to bear down so I let it do what it knew how. The midwife then told me not to push because of the anterior lip (yet another request not respected on my birth plan), so with threats of damaging my cervix and/or my baby I did all I could not to push but without success. She told me not to make the noises (another point on my birth plan) I was making, so I changed them. Then she asked why I was making those noises. I was very frustrated with her at this point and just ignored her. The obstetrician was called back but the anterior lip was still there so with a wave of his hand he declared I had another hour and not to push. (How would he know? I had my money on my body knowing how long it would take.) The midwife suggested drugs (against the birth plan). She had said earlier that if I wanted drugs I had to ask her before hand because she wouldn't be suggesting them to me during the birth and would actively discourage me if I asked for them. I was really starting to think something major must be wrong for all these things to be suggested when I had specifically asked not to be interfered with during the birth. I refused again three times before I believe I am not being given a choice. She even ridiculed the homeopathics I was using. I used the gas but it didn't do a thing – yes, my own hormones were working quite fine and doing their job. There was no opportunity to stay focused on my body birthing.

After my "hour" the midwife announced the obstetrician was caught up with an emergency caesarean and couldn't come so I was not to push until he declared the anterior lip had gone! Exasperated, I said, "If I'm not allowed to push, this baby will be born before I even push!" She suggested that she could check if I liked. For crying out loud, isn't that her job? That was the one vaginal examination I agreed to. It wouldn't have taken Einstein to realise the baby was crowning. "Oh oh oh, the baby's head's right there," she said. "Well yeah, can I push now?"

I firmly believe that how a woman is cared for during her pregnancy and birth has direct impact on the outcome of the birth. If the carer has fear and anxiety about the birth process it will be reflected in her care and transferred to the woman unless she is a stronger woman than I am. As I'd spent the whole birth trying not to push and suddenly I was "allowed" to, I now know I was over-compensating and trying to push too hard. Fortunately at the time I didn't know I was birthing a 4.73kg (10lb 7oz) baby girl because her shoulders proved a little tight and the thought of such a big baby would make anyone doubt themselves. I adopted my upright birthing posture but I was restricted in my movements because of the drip. We got caught in a small space between the bed and the wall, with an anxious midwife keen on interfering – she panicked and started pulling and twisting the baby's head instead of giving us time to birth. I had the entire Birth Centre team in the room: two midwives pulling on her head, and the student doctor holding me down on my back as I tried to get up. (My husband was even told to hold me down, not exactly the supportive role I was expecting him to have.) My saving grace was relaxing and letting them do what they believed was appropriate (even if I didn't) because resisting was only going to make it worse. My daughter Charlotte came out with a crack! The midwife didn't know whether it was the baby or me. I knew it wasn't me.

I was in shock and needed to catch my breath now that it was all over. What had just happened? I never thought I would be grateful that the experience was over. I had really looked forward to the birth and expected to be elated I had a baby, not happy that we were both alive and in one piece. Yet another request from my birth plan denied was to have her examined while I was holding her – she was whisked outside to have tubes stuck down her throat and be prodded and poked. My husband stayed with her but he couldn't touch her because he was given hospital gloves ridiculously too small for him, and why did he need these gloves anyway? Did they think he was going to give her an infection or something? He did a fantastic job of protecting her from any unwanted needles coming her way. While they were outside I was pressured into having an actively managed third stage (again against the birth plan). I couldn't believe it. I just wanted to be able to do something on my own without them interfering. Didn't happen ...

Fortunately my education and training as a chiropractor ensured Charlotte would receive the care she needed to facilitate the healing from such trauma. She had a dislocated shoulder, which was not picked up by the paediatricians, and brainstem damage causing left sided muscle tone weakness that affected her gross motor control. I even enrolled in the International Chiropractic Paediatric Association (ICPA) certification course to advance my skills, having learnt firsthand what can happen in what was considered a "normal birth" by the medical staff.

When I found out I was pregnant with our second baby I wasn't filled with the excitement of being pregnant and the coming birth that I had with the first one, which made me feel very guilty. I was excited about having another baby but just not going through the process again. My first pregnancy was filled with excitement and hormones that made me sky high, while this one was filled with anxiety and worry. I didn't know where to look for care. The Birth Centre still seemed the most closely aligned in philosophy with mine but how had it gone so wrong the first time? I spoke to many professionals connected with birthing and they all suggested I just needed a doula (someone who offers emotional and physical support to a woman and her partner before, during and after childbirth) to be my advocate. I knew a doula, Ingrid Mckenzie, so contacted her. I had met her in prenatal yoga classes and through the Australian Breastfeeding Association; my husband had also met her so I thought she was a good choice. I also thought I should do Calmbirth®, a childbirth preparation course that empowers parents-to-be, women in particular, to take charge of their birthing experience. I had already started the ICPA course by then and completed Jeanne Ohm's Webster Technique Certification. My associate also did the course so we got working on reducing any indications of in-utero constraint. I was doing some business and personal coaching with Dr Sarah Farrant at the time and she guided me through some processes to heal the emotional trauma of the first birth.

I signed up for the Birth Centre program again, but asked for a different midwife, one that a few people had suggested. I went with my birth plan and was very firm about it being adhered to and questioned when it wouldn't be and for what reasons. Ingrid armed me with lots of research material that backed up my own views on certain procedures and tests. It wasn't long before I knew my first birth was going to dictate the care of my second pregnancy. I was very concerned with what had happened with the last birth and I wanted to know why. The more I questioned and the more answers I received, the more I realised I had had a perfectly progressing birth that got interfered with unnecessarily. The midwives at the Birth Centre agreed but it didn't change the way I was going to be cared for; I had a black mark against my name and I couldn't do anything about it, actually three black marks: shoulder dystocia, post-partum haemorrhage and a baby over 4.5 kg (10 lbs) I had to have appointments with an obstetrician and have her agree that I was allowed to birth in the Birth Centre, or not. The first obstetrician agreed but the overruling obstetrician placed unrealistic parameters on me. I had to have a 34 week ultrasound that measured the baby to be on the 50% or less scale before I could stay in the Birth Centre. I know that this test is so inaccurate that no-one ever recommends it or takes it as any indication as to the actual final size of the baby. The 50% or less was just ridiculous because if I had already had a baby well above the 97% mark, I could have another. If she had stated the baby couldn't measure bigger than the first baby then I might have thought her advice had some merit. She tried to intimidate me by saying I was being selfish and didn't have the best interest of my baby at heart and it wasn't all about me. She just didn't seem to hold the idea that if you look after the mother you look after the baby. This was around the time of the large homebirth rally in our capital city and there was a lot of tension between the obstetricians and midwives. It was a political game with the Birth Centre wanting to branch out into homebirthing and the obstetrician trying to prevent it because she wouldn't have control over it and I was getting stuck in the middle. She was clamping down on anyone she could have control over and take from the Birth Centre. I knew if I agreed to this procedure there would only be more hoops to jump through. I was sick of waking every day and preparing myself for a battle with a system hell-bent on interfering when there was no need to. I had to protect myself and my baby from the system. I had to find myself another place to birth.

I had been looking into homebirth as an option for our second birth but thought if I could have my baby in the Birth Centre under my conditions then I would save on the cost of homebirth. As with most things in life, you get what you pay for. As soon as the priority of the baby's and my wellbeing was forefront in our minds, we knew we couldn't stay with the Birth Centre; the dollar cost didn't matter as otherwise the cost was going to be our health, we could see they were not going to be able to provide us with the care we wanted. With the Birth Centre, we were on a one way track to having the same outcome as our first birth and we had to get off that track as fast as possible. (In defence of the Birth Centre and the midwives there, I truly believe they set out to do the best for every woman but they work in a system that is bound by policy and in my situation were not able to compromise. I also believe the medical doctors believe they are doing what they see is the best care and is done with the best of intentions; it just doesn't fit with my understanding of health.) I was stressed and anxious and there was tension building in our relationship.

I started attracting people into my life who were advocates of homebirth: my yoga teacher, my doula, the Calmbirth® teacher, other women in the yoga class, Dr Sarah Farrant, Dr Jeanne Ohm, other chiropractors and their wives. The homebirth rally brought old connections to town who were involved in homebirthing. I just had to take the plunge and commit.

I had heard of Marie Heath, a homebirth midwife, in glowing terms from all angles. She was our only option. As soon as I met her and explained about my first birth and what was happening with the second pregnancy I knew I had the right midwife for me. The major difference to me was she actually practised what she believed in. She believed that I was able to give birth without intervention and that I didn't need the entire hospital to interfere in the delivery of my baby. She was on the same wavelength as me and my views on how the first birth got interfered with. All my new homebirth connections were excited for me too; they knew the value of homebirth from their own experience and supported me in making the decision. Once I committed I was relieved. I stopped stressing and I started to relax and enjoy being pregnant – a niggling pubic pain and pelvic joint pain disappeared; I started communicating with my husband again and we signed up for the Calmbirth® classes privately. I had a lot of emotional baggage to work through to get in the right head space for a homebirth. I got out my pens and got artistic.

As with my first pregnancy, my due date came and went without event. I'd given myself an extra week on my due date after the stress the Birth Centre caused last time so I started to question how "overdue" could I go. Marie called me to my own truth and reassured me that my body knows when the time is right; there is no indication we need to do anything. If I had been at the Birth Centre they would have jumped at the opportunity at my wavering and booked me in for an induction.

I meditated every day on the ability of my body and baby to birth. I made a birthing board with positive affirmations on birth and decorated it with pictures of open flowers. My daily affirmations were: I trust my body, I trust my baby; My body knows how to birth; My baby knows how to birth; My body can't make a baby too big for me to birth; If a woman can give birth in a coma I don't have to do anything; Let my body do what it knows how to do; Just get out of the way and let it happen. I held on to the image shown at one of the Calmbirth® classes of a woman 20 minutes before she gave birth – she was lying on a bed calmly telling herself it is just pressure. This woman had had two prior births that had been nightmares. I held on to the knowledge that it is possible to give birth calmly without interference. I took on the fear-pain-tension message from Calmbirth® about adrenalin causing birth to stall and how to reduce it and promote oxytocin release instead to enhance dilation. Dr Jeanne Ohm had shown us footage of a woman birthing twins in her bathroom and breastfeeding her toddler at the same time in an unattended birth. I just didn't know if this could be me, but I started asking myself the question. Could it? I held onto my belief in my body's ability to birth. I had no other choice; if all those woman had done it then so could I. I held on to the possibility. Dr Sarah Farrant kept reassuring me that the one thing she could guarantee was that the birth would be different to the first one. She focused me on the language I was using that wasn't encouraging like "labour" and "delivery" instead of "birth", and "contractions" instead of "pressure".

The rest of my pregnancy was less eventful. I had been struggling to find the right reading material for this birth preparation but eventually came across a book called *Hands of Love: Seven Steps to the Miracle of Birth* by US chiropractor/doula Carol J Phillips and it just resonated with me. (The writer explains that the outcome of a birth does not make it good or bad; it's not whether it is slow or fast or painful or painless, a birth is just what it is and what you and your baby need it to be.)

Marie's care goes to whoever has the greatest need (i.e. whoever is birthing at the present time gets priority), so at 42 weeks with several cancelled appointments due to other women giving birth, I was feeling a little left out.

I wanted to know when it was my turn to give birth. I had been pre-labouring for a few days but nothing to write home about. Marie was with another woman giving birth so had to cancel my appointment. I called my support friend over because I was feeling miserable and selfish. I wanted it to be my turn to have my baby. She came over straight away and I felt much better. She encouraged me to call Marie and tell her I was niggling, so I did. Marie said I was fine and just pre-labouring and I would see her in a few days. My dad and husband were collecting hay for the garden so were in and out all day with Charlotte. They copped lots of jokes about the men doing the nesting. Dad picked up that I was upset and thought I shouldn't be on my own. He wasn't sold on the homebirth idea and was a little nervous. He called Mum to come over and spend some time with me. We sat on the bed and just chatted. It was a lovely time that I will cherish and remember forever as we don't spend enough time just being together doing nothing.

My doula Ingrid called too. She must have sensed I was in need of support. I asked if she could come over that afternoon, but she said she'd come the next day. I thought tomorrow was too long away; it was my turn to be selfish and ask for what I wanted instead of thinking of others as I usually do. My niggling sensations were not going away this day. I focused on each sensation as if it was opening my cervix. All I could feel was a mild pulling above my pubic bone. I thought I would just try the Calmbirth® techniques, not really thinking I was getting close to birth but it wouldn't hurt anyway just to practise for the real thing. I was sure it was just pre-birth and the real thing was days away. My first birth had been hard, arduous, strenuous work for 10 hours; this felt like a mild period cramp that occurred every ninety minutes or so. I concentrated on the sensations hoping but not believing that this could be what women who don't feel any contractions experience and let it work on my uterus without trying to resist it or put up with it as I had during the first birth. My attitude during my first birth was, I am strong, I can put up with the pain, and I tried to push it away and ignore it. This time I welcomed it and didn't resist. The sensations only went for about 20 seconds and I maintained the conversation only with a slight pause and change of breath. We joked a few times I was probably nine centimetres dilated.

Ingrid left around 4 pm and Mum about 5 pm. The sensations were maybe at closest 20 minutes apart, but not consistent and not increasing in intensity at all. I start to think that maybe this was it and we might have a baby around 1 am. I had a sleep for an hour and woke up for dinner with Rob and Charlotte. Rob noticed the sensations were getting closer together and asked when the last one was. I had been asleep so didn't really know but thought maybe one had woken me up. I said he should keep track as I was tuning out of the world and into my body. I didn't want to be distracted by observing my body, I just wanted to be in my body and let it do what it needed to and not get in the way of the process. I didn't want timing and watching the clock to be my gauge; I was only going to take notice of what my body was telling me. After dinner he said they were about 10 minutes apart. Ok, I was now convinced it would be tonight. I was in no hurry to call Marie because I knew she was still with the other woman birthing and I was expecting to be like this for hours yet.

Around 7 pm we were putting Charlotte to bed and she was asking for a breastfeed. Not exactly what I was planning to be doing at the time but thought it was better to have her settled and in bed so we could get ready for the birth, and the nipple stimulation would help the oxytocin production anyway. I lay on our bed feeding Charlotte while Rob (my husband) gently stroked my back to encourage endorphin release. I still thought I was being premature in starting the Calmbirth® techniques but thought what the heck it can't hurt. I asked Rob to run his fingers through my hair but he just got the hair in my eyes so I directed him back to stroking my back. When I stopped focusing on the pulling sensation and tried to ignore it, it actually felt worse, and the more I focused on it the less it bothered me. I had a moment's thought about how frustrating the whole "pre-birth" process was and that I just wanted the birth to start for real. I was annoyed with myself that I had to work so hard at staying calm. I could sense if I didn't stay calm it could easily take over and get out of control.

I quickly stopped myself from entertaining those thoughts as they were not going to help me. (In hindsight this was my transition) Rob said the sensations were five to six minutes apart now – he was just judging by the slight change in the depth of my breath. We quickly put Charlotte to bed at 7.20 pm.

I thought I had just stirred things up by breastfeeding and wanted to get in the bath to relax and settle down. I was thinking we had time; we'll get ourselves ready, get the support team back, get the pool ready and settle in to make an evening of it. I went to the toilet and had a mild sensation to want to push. I thought this was interesting because last time it wasn't something I could choose to do or not. I trusted my body and decided since I didn't have to push then I would not and I'd let my body do what it knew how to do.

Rob ran the bath and called Marie – it was 7.29 pm. She was heading to the hospital with the woman she had been with all day so she said she'd call a stand-in midwife. Rob rang Ingrid and said things have progressed and we'll call you back when we know for sure it's happening. What part of "it is happening now" he didn't understand I'm not sure. Rob went to the lounge room to tidy up and set up the birth pool. I couldn't get comfortable in the bath. I couldn't lie down. I was on all fours and the water didn't reach my belly. I then realised it was happening right now, not in a few hours but right now, and fast. I called Rob back to the bathroom, "It's happening right now." I had a hot flush race down my back which called for a cold washer (in hindsight probably my adrenalin surge). The stand-in midwife, Georgia, who said she had a call from Marie to check on me, rang. I didn't want Rob to put me on the phone as I was so calm and nothing was going to make me otherwise. Midwives always ask to speak to the woman to gauge what stage she is at and I knew if I spoke to her she wouldn't think the birth was imminent. Anyway, Rob put me on and I calmly accepted her offer to come over. I should have screamed, "I'm having the baby right now", but I thought better of it. She was on her way. Rob called Ingrid back and told her it was happening right now. She was half an hour away. I had an overwhelming urge to bear down and I felt my membranes pop. I breathed deep and hard and told myself not to push so hard; it will happen on its own. I can feel the head! I realise we are going to have the baby on our own. Stay calm. Rob said, "It's ok; it's gone back up now," and I said: "Yeah, but it's coming in the next push!" Stay calm. We got Ingrid back on the phone as we didn't have Georgia's number. She said she could get there in 20 minutes but knew she wasn't going to make it. She suggested I get out of the bath, because at this point, if I stay in the bath the baby will dive bomb into the water. I slid out of the bath and onto the mat. Stay calm. I asked Rob what he could see and he replied one after the other as each emerged – forehead, eyebrows, eyes, cheekbones, nose, mouth. I took a breath and reflected on my previous birth and how different this one had been; there is no way the shoulders are getting stuck this time, it's just been too different. At 7.45 pm Rob took the catch of his life.

"It's another girl," he said, I double-check – he forgot to look when Charlotte was born and almost presumed she was a boy. Oh my gosh! We did it, and on our own! And oh so easy. Wow! I held my crying baby girl, thinking, "That's good; that means she's breathing; everything is ok." Now that's how you're supposed to come into the world: no pushing, no pulling, just letting it all happen.

We quickly woke Charlotte who had been in bed for only 20 minutes. She excitedly declared "Bay-be" and pointed out all her body parts and where my breasts were for mi-mi. We retired to the bedroom. Ingrid arrived 10 minutes later and suggested giving a little push and I birth the placenta. Georgia the substitute midwife arrived 10 minutes later, surprised we already had the baby and the placenta. Ingrid was on hand to help me with baby-led attachment, guiding me in allowing Eleanor to self-attach – but she needed no guidance. I even had an ice-cream in bed just because I felt like it and because I could. I'd had a homebirth. I could do what I liked!

We called Marie who was on her way to the operating theatre with the other woman. She was blown away by the birth and how we'd done it by ourselves and so quickly without fuss. With all the pressure from the medical field we turned around a difficult challenging experience and made it an exceptional one. Marie called in at 6 am the following day to check on us before going home to sleep. Eleanor was 4.4 kg (9lb 11oz) our "little" baby, lighter than her sister but longer at 58cm. No stitches were required.

Dad was fascinated by the placenta. As he walked in it was in the laundry and the midwife told him it gets eaten in some cultures so he and Mum spend the next few days looking up placenta recipes on the internet. (We didn't eat the placenta; it was planted beneath a peach tree in our yard.)

Everyone involved in the homebirth supported me to stand up for my rights as a birthing woman and not to be railroaded by a medical system run on fear. We can feel proud we did it our way, the way we knew was possible and the way it can be done. I am now a passionate advocate for homebirth and can appreciate the difference first hand. Knowledge is empowerment and knowing first hand the importance of getting the support team right for you and the tools to manage birth is life changing. I can't thank everyone enough.

My two birth experiences reflect the way health care is practised in Australia and most of the developed world and what can be achieved with a chiropractic philosophy of health. The health care industry is run in a way that removes responsibility of health outcomes from the individual involved and places it onto the practitioner. This creates a situation where blame or credit is placed on the practitioner providing the care for the health of the individual and thus decisions are made in fear of litigation and in mistrust of the human body. Once you are free to take responsibility for your own health outcomes, as seen through chiropractic care, an individual owns their own health and they are able to step forward to a new level of life, and amazing transformations are seen.

CHAPTER 17

"The hardest people to convince they are at retirement age are children at bedtime."

Shannon Fife

No More Sleepless Nights! No More Crying Babies!

By Sandy Clark

When a couple are thinking of having children, the subject of a crying baby rarely comes up as an important issue to understand or consider. As the couple's pregnancy continues and birth stories start to come to light from other mothers and friends, the focus is usually on labour and breathing and just holding the new little life that is growing inside this mother-to-be. There are parenting classes and help is all around, but until this new life actually cries inconsolably and nothing you do seems to make one scrap of difference, do you ever even think of colic?

As a chiropractor and a parent I do and it's one of the many reasons parents bring their children to see me. My aim is always to address all of the contributing factors and then offer some possible solutions.

So what is colic? Essentially, colic is a description not a diagnosis and it describes a child who is unsettled and crying without being able to be consoled for at least three hours in a day, for more than three days of a week and for three weeks continuously. It is not a definitive diagnosis that will answer why the child is crying or what can be done about the crying child to help settle them down, however this 3x3x3 of crying, known as the Wessel criteria, is a test tool or score sheet used by health care providers to assess if a child is presenting with colic-like symptoms.

The reason colic is so important to understand is because it affects the child and everyone surrounding the child. Let's start with some facts: two thirds of all hospital admissions for children under the age of six months are due to the child crying inconsolably; 56% of these children have diarrhoea, reflux or a urinary tract infection and only 5% of these are serious enough to require further examination. Colic represents 10% of these hospital admissions and all of the associated conditions could be assessed by a chiropractor and can usually be found by asking a few basic questions during the initial examination. Most, if not all, children in a hospital setting who have a diagnosis of colic are generally sent home, so it is important to have your chiropractor assess your child if they are crying, to find out what is the most likely cause of the crying.

So you now have a child with colic-type symptoms of crying, irritability, poor sleeping habits, hard to settle, hard to feed and generally needing to be held. As a chiropractor, my main concerns are how the family is coping as individuals and as a whole. The bond between parents and a child has been seen to improve every aspect of a child's health and the best way to bond with a newborn is through skin-to-skin contact as often as possible. As for health issues, if the research is to be believed, there is no one thing that makes or breaks colic; however, chiropractors are looking for the hidden causes behind the symptoms that are driving the child to cry excessively and be generally irritable. Why is this child's nervous system wired to produce a symptom of crying as the only response and why, even when all other issues (dirty nappy, too hot, too cold, need a feed, need a poo …) have been taken care of, does the response seem to go on for hours or more.

In published research regarding colic, its causes, what may aggravate it, and what can be done about it, the majority of research is looking at what is happening with the child right now and while this is a crucial part of managing the symptoms of colic it doesn't address how the problem starts. The published research by chiropractors shows that chiropractic helps with colic; however it doesn't touch on what most chiropractors are assessing.

Here are a few of the possible things that a chiropractor will be looking for and be able to help with, either by assessing the mother during her pregnancy or by assessing the colicky child:

- **KISS syndrome (Kinematic Imbalance and Suboccipital Strain syndrome)** – where, either in utero or during labour and the birthing process, excessive flexing forward or extending backwards of the neck has occurred which has then strained the muscles at the base of the skull. This muscle strain causes inflammation to the surrounding delicate blood vessels and nerves, which has been seen to cause torticollis type conditions where a child is unable to fully turn their head to one or both sides.

- **Intra-uterine constraint** – where the growing foetus has been restricted while in utero, which is thought to produce long labour times, poor baby positioning, plagiocephaly (a flattening of the baby's skull), start the KISS syndrome, and usually results in lower back pain during pregnancy and a painful labour. The restriction is usually caused by tension in the ligaments that support the pelvis and hold the uterus in place.

- **Birth trauma** – from a chiropractic point of view and for most mothers who have given birth (and for any of us second-hand observers ... fathers) all births are traumatic, a lot of births have KISS syndrome associated with them and if your child is delivered by an obstetrician then the likelihood of associated trauma to the child's cervical spine has been shown in published research to be increased.

- Then there is **GER (gastroesophageal reflux)** – which is simply a new way of describing reflux, and the latest research that is being done is showing that 50% of reflux is non-acidic, which answers why medication for acid reflux only works 50% of the time. The misdiagnosis of reflux and colic has led to poor management and a prolonging of the problem for mother and the child.

- There are no statistics as yet that can support this next theory – however, if the mother has lots of digestion issues during her pregnancy, or has gestational diabetes, or allergic reactions during pregnancy that are worse or new compared to when she wasn't pregnant, then the likelihood of her child having colic is somewhat increased. As well as allergies in the child or intolerances to whey (milk protein), **chiropractic research shows that removing the pressure on the nerves at the base of the skull by way of specific adjustment can help relieve the symptoms of colic in up to 92% of cases.**

There are a number of neurological responses involved with a crying child and their seemingly unresponsiveness to being soothed or cared for. All neurological responses (or reflexes) are what a chiropractor tests for and can help to correct in all children. The most important reflexes in a child are called primitive reflexes and these are there from the moment a child is born and are slowly over-written by higher brain functions as the child ages. These reflexes and the over-writing process that occurs in the brain can be tested during a normal visit to your chiropractor and are used as a way of assessing the effectiveness of the adjustment at each visit; however, depending on the child and the reflex responses involved, the adjustments may need to be repeated over a number of weeks in order to change the reflex pattern.

As every child is different, there is no one way that is right or the best that a mother, father or carer can do except to be patient and consistent with their child and allow the time it takes to get to know the child's ideals as far as being cared for go. There is no right answer for every colicky child; just rule out everything that could be going on that may make the child cry by taking them to a chiropractor so they can help you understand allergic reactions, intolerances to whey (milk protein), diarrhoea, reflux or other neurological causes, and then allow the child to heal and grow, naturally

CHAPTER 18

"The doctor of the future will give no medicine,
but will interest her or his patients in the care
of the human frame, in a proper diet, and in the
cause and prevention of disease."

Thomas A. Edison

Family Wellbeing

By Ed Groenhart

Should chiropractors be as central a part of everyday family health as dentists? I think so because, just like dentists, chiropractors have a preventative role at the core of their health philosophy. In this chapter we'll be looking at the role chiropractic can play in helping your family stay fit and healthy and living with more life in their years. I'll be reviewing how stress has such a vital role at all stages of life, even at our birth, and how it is becoming an ever more evident cause of modern health issues in the so-called developed world.

So, what is stress? Well, there are three stresses: chemical (toxins), physical (trauma), and emotional (thoughts). DD Palmer, founder of the chiropractic profession, coined the term "The Three Ts", which is far easier to remember. Stresses lead to symptoms (aches and pains) via overload of the body's ability to cope with stress and strain. Think of it as the body adapting to strain, like an iron girder bending under the strain of ever-larger weights placed upon it until, finally, something snaps. Symptoms are our body's red light indicating damage has been done, and we need to heed them until healing has completed.

I mentioned above that our own birth is the first stress. Birth trauma is the first challenge the fragile infant body has to overcome. This is not to say that birth is inevitably a horrible process for mother and child. On the contrary, a natural birth is a beautiful (if, unfortunately these days, uncommon) event. However, with any problematic presentation of the child, such as breech, we have potential issues. Further physical stresses can be placed on the infant with the use of ventouse (vacuum), forceps or medication to alter the natural flow of the process. As well as any medication, chemical stresses are passed from mother to baby in the form of stress hormones. The infant's system is easily overwhelmed, leading to adaptive change in body structure and function.

Studies as far back as 1969, and later in the 1980s, found that traumatic birth methods can be the cause of spinal injury, spinal misalignment and cranial distortions, which may often escape diagnosis. If these spinal injuries are never corrected, the baby's ability to adapt to the new (external) environment is hampered. The importance of a developing child being free from nerve interference cannot be understated.

In 1993, a medical researcher named Gottlieb stated in one of his articles that: "Birth trauma remains an under-publicised and therefore an under-treated problem. There is a need for further documentation and especially more studies directed towards prevention."

Fortunately, the evidence pointing towards the importance of chiropractic in childhood is growing at a rapid rate. Studies in the past 20 years have strongly pointed to chiropractic having a role at the head of childhood health, and why not? Would any parent want to resort to routine medication or even surgery ahead of what is an extremely safe, conservative approach? Danish studies on colic, Canadian studies on childhood asthma, and Australian research on recurrent and chronic ear infections all strongly point to chiropractic's role in managing (and perhaps even preventing) these common childhood ailments.

Fortunately, evidence is being obtained to show that chiropractic may have a role in childhood health, and why not? Would any parent not want to know of a conservative approach, particularly if medication or surgery were undesired options? Cranial techniques and massage may have favourable effects on colic, and forms of manipulation such as Osteopathic Manipulative Therapy (OMT) may help asthma as well as ear infections, although this is less clear. As with many conditions, more and better research needs to be done; however, it is starting to happen. As I mention a little later, this is not only applicable to chiropractic.

Of course, as we go into adolescence and adulthood, an increasing amount of time is spent studying and working, often at a desk. Modern, "developed world" sedentary lifestyles mean that although strenuous physical work, in the form of manufacturing and agricultural work, has decreased, another form of physical trauma, in the form of repetitive stress injuries, has increased. Additionally, chemical and emotional stress has increased as life has become less naturally challenging (there are no sabre-toothed tigers chasing us any more), but unnatural challenges (fast-paced lives, sterile environments, chemical pollution) have increased.

So why don't chiropractors see young and old members of the family? We see dentists for checks to our teeth, why not chiropractors for checks to our spines, posture and resulting general healthy function. We've looked at many of the features of chiropractic but how can it prove itself in modern healthcare? It's true that chiropractic is a young and growing healing art. The underlying tenet of chiropractic maintains that balancing the body through its core, both structurally and functionally, leads to changes in body balance, both structurally and functionally. As the spine houses the most vulnerable part of the Master Control System (the central nervous system), it makes sense to protect this area and ensure that the whole system is able to operate free of interference. This creates an opportunity for *everyone* to achieve their full potential through natural means, without the need for drugs or surgery, as part of an overall healthy lifestyle. This is the holistic approach of chiropractic; one that is by no means novel but has been overlooked by many other professions in pursuit of the elusive "quick fix" that modern society demands. Unfortunately, all too often these approaches are a misleading quick fix that never delivers fully.

The chiropractic model is free of drugs and surgery. As I said before, does any parent want a "drugged" child? Is a child who only sleeps through the night due to medication a healthy, happy child? As for taking a medical opinion as gospel, the British Medical Journal in 1991 reported: "Only 15% of medical interventions are supported by solid scientific evidence". Considering medicine is the basis of our health systems, surely this is a sobering statistic for anyone who takes medicines without first reading the label? It is true that medicine has a stronger role in healthcare at present, but this has not always been the case, and public opinion has a role to play in the type of healthcare most widely available.

Hang on though, aren't many problems hereditary? Arthritis is one example that is often thought to be almost entirely hereditary, if not completely unavoidable in later life. In actual fact, there are many forms of arthritis, but by far the most common, and most easy to prevent with appropriate lifestyle modifications, is osteoarthritis, or OA for short. This is the single biggest reason for one of the most expensive common orthopaedic operations, the hip replacement.

Osteoarthritis was first shown to develop in rats with a limb immobilised in plaster. The lack of exercise/movement and flexibility led to arthritic changes in the joints, leading researches to realise that this is the most important factor determining the likelihood of getting OA in joints in the body. The rats weren't left to live a normal life, and then found to get OA! The affected joints were merely immobilised – a strong signal indeed to today's sedentary younger generations that, as sure as night follows day, an arthritis epidemic is emerging as they become less and less active.

It is true that there are many genetic forms of all sorts of degenerative disease processes, no doubt including OA, but genes are often only expressed when placed in an environment that allows that gene expression to flourish; that is, an environment filled with the appropriate stresses.

Chiropractic works *with* the body, allowing for nature's constraints, helping each person, old or (especially) young, to achieve their full potential. Chiropractors initially approach everyone the same way – with a broad approach, looking at that person's history and lifestyle in detail. Once all the evidence is gathered, they will go about advising on both preventive measures and on **The 5 Pillars of a Healthy Lifestyle:**

1. **Sleep and Adequate Rest**

2. **Exercise,** both in general, and specific to any problems (see also Sports chapter). Chiropractors will often recommend a "core" exercise in order to promote recovery and prevent recurrence, such as Pilates, Tai Chi or yoga.

3. **Diet** – Hydration and Nutrition (See *Changing Habits Changing Lives* by Cyndi O'Meara for more details.)

4. **Positive Mental Attitude** has a role to play in both recovery from injury and health promotion. There is increasing evidence that there is an emotional root to many chronic back problems, especially in females.

5. **A Fully Functioning Body,** completely aligned and fully controlled by its Master Control System (the central nervous system).

Why do chiropractors go into detail with their assessment, only to give general recommendations? The history is vital! It is the history of current and past problems, combined with family medical history and both current and past stresses, that allows appraisal of the stress load on each individual body. Making appropriate, effective changes to lifestyle helps to get the best long-term results. Remember, we are looking to not only treat the current problems but also prevent future problems by nipping them in the bud where possible, just as a dentist does. Chiropractic has recognised that it's not always possible to completely cure or eliminate illness and disease, but we can arm families with the basic knowledge to make healthy choices and lead healthier and therefore happier and more fulfilled lifestyles.

CHAPTER 19

"An ounce of prevention is worth a pound of cure."

Benjamin Franklin

Active Kids

By Linda Balazic-Vandenberg

A ll parents want their children to grow up and achieve the most they can out of life: to be healthy, do well at school, be successful in sports or just excel in life. Giving children a loving environment, a healthy diet and exercise are essential, but most parents are unaware that chiropractic care can be added into their family's regular health routine to give their children a proactive natural way to improve their health and wellness. Chiropractic recognises that the body has an innate ability to heal itself, on the condition that the nervous system is functioning optimally.

Unique, effective drug-free approach

Chiropractic teaches a child to look at the underlying causes when the body is not functioning at a high level and not to just cover up the warning signs (symptoms) our body gives us, by popping pills such as pain killers. It's important we teach our children that the answer is not to look in the medicine cabinet, but that health comes from within. Our body is precious and we have to work towards looking after it, because this body and brain are the only ones we are given.

Chiropractic has a unique, drug-free approach and its success is driven by client satisfaction and people telling their family and friends about their experiences.

The positive effects of chiropractic care vary from child to child. I hear parents excitedly talking in the waiting room comparing how the health of their children has improved – from being more calm and able to concentrate better at school, having better posture, to better rested babies who feed better and don't get sick as often so their use of medication and antibiotics has reduced, just to name a few.

Our profession has been working towards validating these results we see daily in practice. Much of the positive evolution of chiropractic can be ascribed to a quarter-century-long research effort, although we still have a way to go. Chiropractic is a young profession – in 2005 it celebrated its 110th anniversary – however it is the largest, most regulated, and best recognised of the professions that have traditionally functioned outside mainstream medical institutions.[1]

Why treat babies?

When people see me adjusting babies and children, I often get asked, "Why do you treat babies?" How can children develop problems with their backs or nerves?

This is a very good question, and to answer it we have to think right back to the beginning of life. The first physical stressors may be seen in the first trimester of pregnancy when the foetus is in a malposition, causing in-utero constraint.[2] The infant in the breech position is also more likely to have a hip dislocation[3], mandibular asymmetry (crooked or uneven jaw), and postural distortion (bad posture).

The delivery often causes trauma to the spine and possible subluxations (nerve interference).[4] The immense compression and then stretching of the baby's delicate spine involved in even normal delivery can cause damage. Difficult labour, forceps, vacuum extraction, and Caesarean section exacerbate the situation.

Excessive crying, arching of the back, uneven movement of the arms and legs, an uneven skull, and not settling, are all early signs that there may be problems with a baby's nervous system.[5]

What can cause problems in a child's nervous system?

In the next few years of life we must consider:

- Falls head first from a high place such as a change table or bed
- Baby walker injuries
- Car accidents
- Hundreds of falls as toddlers learn to walk and run. I remember I always had a collection of bruises I was very proud of from falls off my bike and out of trees. In my practice, children falling down stairs at home are common, even under close supervision; it only takes looking away for a split second.

As children reach school age, habitually carrying heavy school bags on one shoulder can cause spinal problems. Backpacks are best, and must be worn correctly. Lack of exercise and working at computers or at a desk, playing video games or watching TV for long periods with poor posture can also be unhealthy for the growing body.

The body has to continuously deal with these physical stresses, but also emotional and chemical stresses too. Chemical stressors can include an unbalanced diet high in processed foods or low in fresh fruit and vegetables, air pollution, chemicals used in the home such as cleaning products, and allergies or intolerances to certain foods.

Emotional stress can include problems in the family home, and pressures at school such as learning difficulties or bullying, or the loss of a loved one. When several types of stress build up during someone's life, the natural resistance of the body gradually becomes less, then the ability of the body to adapt and compensate decreases. The human body is very resilient and I'm constantly amazed at how it deals with what we subject it to on a daily basis, but if the stressors overcome the amount a body can cope with and physically compensate for, the body will start to function below an optimal level. This can cause structural changes, especially in the spine and the pelvis, and these changes can disturb the balance of the nervous system. Over time this may lead to acute symptoms and illness which, left untreated, may become chronic conditions.

One study examined a group of apparently healthy children and found that 15.8% had cervical subluxations (neck problems) and 40% had pelvic subluxations.[6] So pain is not an accurate indicator of underlying problems.

The conventional medical model encourages parents to bring in their children when they show signs and symptoms of illness, but not to return when they have recovered. People also come to chiropractors for physical complaints; in this sense, chiropractic is a way to restore nervous system function so the body can heal itself. It is important though that "healthy" people use chiropractic as a preventative, having regular check-ups to be sure that changes in the nervous system can be diagnosed and corrected at an early stage. This could never be more important than in a child. Hannon SM[7] concluded that it is plausible that chiropractic care may be of benefit to every function of the body and have the potential for long-term, overall health benefit to those receiving chiropractic care.

There was a comparative study of the health status of children raised under the health care models of chiropractic and allopathic medicine.[8] This was a very interesting study involving two hundred paediatricians and two hundred chiropractors that were randomly selected. Each participant was sent a survey to determine whether there were any differences in the health status of their respective children.

In essence, the study was comparing the health of children raised under two different health care models: on the one hand the medical model of health and on the other the chiropractic model.

The results showed nearly 43% of the medical children had suffered from tonsillitis, compared to less than 27% of the chiropractic children. Lower antibiotic use and lower incidence of disease, especially ear infections, was reported in the chiropractic children. If the chiropractic children did get measles, rubella or mumps, it was reported that the diseases were quite mild compared to those exhibited by their classmates. Wow! Is that ever great news!

A chiropractor is a specialist in stabilising the spinal cord by finding and correcting interference in the nervous system. I've lost count of the thousands of times I've assessed a client and located a subluxation or area of tension in the body and asked if it's tender, and the answer is, "Yes. How do you always manage to find the right spots without me telling you where they are?" It is extensive chiropractic training and experience that helps in treating babies when they cannot give you feedback.

Good posture

Good posture is important. I have often walked past a hunched-over elderly person in the street and immediately realised that I was not standing as straight as I could, and quickly straightened my spine. Do you do that? A person's posture gives chiropractors a good indication of the health of the spine, muscles and nervous system, and good posture is particularly important for growing children.

For Sally*, a 15-year-old girl I see in practice, standing straight is painful as is sitting at school, so her concentration and learning is affected. Her problems developed because she is tall and has to stoop to talk to her shorter friends, and the desks at her school are non-adjustable and are too small for her. But with regular adjustments she is pain free and her posture is now greatly improved.

Chiropractic has been shown to improve the posture of clients.[9] In children, it is better to correct the problems before poor posture leads to bad habits. It is easier to deal with a 10-year-old with postural problems than someone who comes in at 40 years old and has a lifetime of bad habits to undo. Misalignments from even minor trauma should be checked and corrected if needed, because, "Unless the injuries are treated, by the time these children have reached adulthood, the compensatory asymmetries will almost certainly have become fixed and themselves require treatment."[10]

Brain development in children

The first ten years of life see the biggest changes in brain development that will determine important healthy brain patterns and connections (neural plasticity). Chiropractic helps maximise a child's neural plasticity[11] by locating and correcting areas in the body where the nervous system is compromised; the brain is then best able to manage and control the functions of the entire body.

One child I treated whilst practising in the Netherlands stands out in my mind – a young boy called Martin*. He was having problems keeping up with his schoolmates with his reading and writing and was about to be put down a level at school. His parents were so pleased with his chiropractic care because within two months he sat his next test and his writing skills had improved so much the teacher thought he cheated and made him do it again – she was astounded by the results because apart from the chiropractic care, no other variables had been changed. The teacher noticed he found it easier to focus and concentrate. Also, looking at the bigger picture, he loved going to school again as his confidence grew, and he stayed in his normal class with his peers.

It may be many years before we fully understand how the brain really works and have sufficient scientific data to back up these cases seen in practice;

however, research studies[12,13] suggest that chiropractic adjustment may enhance brain function. This is very exciting work which, as our technology continues to evolve, will give us a window into observing how brain activity changes as a result of spinal care. The results indicated that adjustment of the neck could have a powerful effect on the function of the brain.

What do chiropractors do to help your child?

The chiropractic corrections, what we call "adjustments", are very specific and are applied to the areas of your child's body that have shown to be areas of nerve interference. These adjustments are extremely gentle and can be applied by different techniques. Personally, I use a light index finger contact and hold for a short period of time, with a quick release. It's as gentle as the pressure you can easily withstand on your eyeball or you use to test the firmness of a tomato. Sometimes an instrument called an activator is used to help to achieve the same light touch. The children generally enjoy the experience and, once old enough, jump up on the table to be first. Advice and ongoing encouragement is given to parents regarding relevant lifestyle advice for their family, including posture, back packs, nutrition, sleeping positions and exercise.

Every chiropractor is qualified to treat children. There are many ongoing paediatric chiropractic seminars additional to the core university training for practitioners to stay abreast of all the latest techniques and research. There are also fully accredited Masters of Chiropractic Paediatrics degrees, which increase a chiropractor's knowledge and competence to the highest level. Your chiropractor will be happy to discuss their level of training and if your child has a condition outside the scope of chiropractic, an appropriate external referral will be made.

Chiropractic care is a rewarding experience. It is an essential part of a preventative, natural, healthy lifestyle. It encourages your family to be proactive and prioritise health choices to look after the one and only body we are given. In the years to come, your children will thank you for it!

(*Patients names changed to protect confidentiality.)

CHAPTER 20

"The future depends on what we do in the present."

Mahatma Gandhi

Learning Difficulties – A Common Sense Approach

By Rachael Talbot

An increasing number of parents are taking their children with common learning disorders/disabilities such as ADHD (Attention Deficit Hyperactivity Disorder), ADD (Attention Deficit Disorder), Dyspraxia, Dyslexia, and those on the Autistic Spectrum (including Asperger's Syndrome), to see chiropractors.

Although they are often viewed as separate conditions, there is considerable overlap between these disorders. Obsessive Compulsive Disorder (OCD) and Tourette's Syndrome are also commonly associated with this spectrum. Many of these children show a combination of symptoms. Neurologically, many of these traits can be traced to two key areas of the brain – the pre-frontal cortex and the cerebellum – and as discussed by Pauc (2005) for this reason all of these conditions can be considered together under the banner of Learning Disorders (Developmental Delay).[1]

Regardless of which diagnosis these children have, the picture is often similar. They often struggle at school, their concentration levels are deemed lower than average and they are underperforming academically, even though many of them are extremely intelligent. They find it hard to sit still and are easily distracted. Physically these children can be poorly coordinated and struggle with sport. They are often the "clumsy" kids who never get picked for sports teams and can be the subject of bullying. Many of them also have a whole host of what could be termed "psychological conditions" including depression, anxiety, low self esteem, obsessive compulsive disorder and Tourette's Syndrome (involuntary tics or spoken words). A good number of these children are also hypersensitive to environmental stimuli such as touch or noise or smells; when present, this can cause considerable distress. Already you can see that this is a long list of symptoms, and each child will display their own unique combination of these.

Medically, the approach that receives most media attention is Ritalin and other drugs from the same class. Ritalin is an amphetamine, which is the same class of drug as the recreational drug Speed. It is a stimulant and has become one of the main lines of treatment for ADHD. Clinically, Ritalin can be successful in improving concentration, but there are increasing concerns about its safety and the long term effects. Other drugs that have been used with some success include anti-depressant medications. However, some children cannot tolerate these drugs or do not respond, and many parents do not want to medicate their children. Drugs don't address the cause but focus on modifying the symptoms, and the long-term effects of doing this are not yet fully understood. Detailed discussion of these drugs is beyond the scope of this chapter.

Other approaches that may be offered include Cognitive Behavioural Therapy (CBT), psychotherapy, social skill training and parenting skills, all with varying success.

So where does chiropractic fit into all of this? And what does chiropractic have to do with behaviour and thoughts? After all, pain is the reason most people consult a chiropractor in the 21st century.

Chiropractic was founded on the scientific fact that the body is self-healing and that the nervous system coordinates healing within the body.

> *For more than a hundred years now, chiropractors have been helping individuals to achieve optimum health through working with the function of the spine.*

Chiropractic is all about the nervous system. It is argued that the nervous system is the most important system within the human body because it provides a central role in coordinating health. We perceive our world through our nervous system (eyes, ears, touch, etc). It also coordinates our immune system, digestion, thoughts and actions, so to express optimal health we need our nervous system to be functioning optimally.

Chiropractors can evaluate nervous system function through a number of different methods including spinal function, posture, range of motion (global and segmental), surface EMG (electromyography), neurological testing, balance and coordination.

Clinically, the following may be observed with children on the Learning Disorder Spectrum:

- Lack of flexibility in their spines
- Restrictions to the upper neck

- Restrictions to the lower back and pelvis

- Poor balance

- Poor hand-eye coordination

- Problems tracking with the eyes (following a moving object using the eyes without moving the head)

- Problems accommodating (bringing the eyes together in a coordinated manner)

- Poor posture

When the history of the child is investigated further we commonly hear a combination of the following, some of which are in the past, some of which may be still present:

- Difficult or traumatic birth (e.g. an emergency c-section, forceps or vacuum delivery)

- Bad sleeper

- Visible asymmetry as baby

  - Looks only to one side

  - Favours one arm or leg

  - Favours one breast when feeding

  - Bald spot on back of head

- Hypersensitive in neck region

- Twin or triplet

- Didn't crawl, or crawled asymmetrically or commando style

- Delayed motor and/or language skills

- Walked very early (and didn't crawl)

- Chronic ear infections

- Food intolerances

This list is not all inclusive. You may see it and respond: "Well loads of children have these things in their history." Yes, that's true. But the latest data from the USA suggests that 3–10%[3] of children and 1–6% of adults suffer from Learning Disorders/Disabilities, so what we're talking about is common.

Many of the symptoms and conditions listed above respond well to chiropractic care, so if your child is exhibiting any of these you may be well advised to consult a chiropractor with an interest in Paediatrics. Other chapters address many of these issues.

But what happens if you already have a child with a learning disorder. There is a growing body of research to support the use of chiropractic for children with learning disorders and associated symptoms. As early as 1974, Walton reported improvements in these children using chiropractic methods to be 24% more effective than the drug therapy of the day.

A blinded, controlled study reported over 71% improvement in behaviour and 57% improvement in parentally observed hyperactivity in a group of seven subjects.[2] A recent study from Switzerland of nine adults showed significant improvements of the symptoms of Attention Deficit Hyperactivity Disorder in all participants.[3]

An increasing number of case studies in recent years show partial or complete resolution of the symptoms of ADHD[4-11] in both adults and children.

Biederman (2005) discusses the link between birth and restriction to the upper neck region. He carried out research on children in a school specialising in learning difficulties and noted that where children had a history suggestive of upper cervical strain, these children showed cognitive improvement after spinal manipulation.

A further study linked trauma and ADHD, and observed that where developmental delay is thought to be secondary to trauma and associated sensory-motor impairment, chiropractic may be successfully employed in the treatment of dyslexia, dyspraxia, learning disabilities and ADHD.[12]

So why would chiropractic have these effects? The spinal column is a physical window to the nervous system encasing the spinal cord. The brain receives information from the whole body via the nervous system and all the nerves must first pass through the spinal cord. There are numerous chiropractic techniques, but they share a goal of improving spinal function so that messages can flow between the body and the brain.

The two key areas of the brain that are especially important in learning disorders are the cerebellum and the pre-frontal cortex. The cerebellum has long been accepted as key for motor learning and coordination. It also appears that it is involved in almost all functions of the brain including control of motor, sensory, autonomic, cognitive, emotional and behavioural responses.[13] The majority of sensory input from the spine to the brain comes from the upper cervical spine. It is thought that the use of chiropractic to restore function to the neck can significantly improve the input the brain gets from the body and hence improves the function of the cerebellum. This, in turn, improves balance, coordination and spacial awareness, and also our coordination of emotions and behaviours. As many of these children are immature socially, this has huge implications for developing friendships and confidence. Research from the USA also showed that a proportion of children with ADHD also have convergence disorder, or, put simply, the inability to focus the eyes for sustained periods of time.[14] The cerebellum plays a crucial role in convergence.

The frontal lobes are involved in motor function, concentration, problem solving, spontaneity, memory, language, initiation, judgement, impulse control and social and sexual behaviour.[15] Injury or lack of development can result in loss or reduction in any of the behaviours associated with these functions and can also see pseudo-depression or pseudo-psychopathic behaviours develop where injury is sufficient.[16] Function of the frontal lobes is closely linked to motor ability. Activation of spinal pathways through chiropractic adjustment is believed to activate the frontal lobe and improve both motor and cognitive/ emotional/behaviour function.[17] There is also chiropractic research which suggests that improving function of the spine can have an impact on how the frontal lobes perform.[18]

There is a strong link between motor function and executive function. This is one reason why exercise is so important in developing and sustaining neurological function. Practically we can understand this best if we look at how exercise improves our sense of wellbeing. We often feel better physically and emotionally after exercise. If there is a magic bullet to better health, it's exercise (it appears protective to the heart, endocrine system, immune system, etc). During exercise the spine moves, stimulating the nervous system. It also pumps more blood around the body delivering more oxygen and glucose to the brain. Exercise is an essential part of healing for children with learning disorders, increasing the ability to concentrate and focus attention. Lack of exercise can add to the problem.

The research of Candace Pert links spinal function to our emotions.[19] This supported the work of Blanks (1997), which showed improvements in emotional and mental function and stress handling in response to chiropractic care[20], all areas of which are commonly problems in these children.

To fully address the health of your child, although chiropractic provides an excellent baseline because it improves the function of the nervous system, which coordinates the expression of health; you may also need to address your child's diet and their exercise profile.

Many of these children are fussy and self-select their diet, predominantly to one of processed carbohydrates and sugary drinks. This diet does not support healthy development of the nervous system. However challenging, it is essential that children eat a balanced diet of fruit, vegetables, grains and protein and that they remain well hydrated (ideally from water). Many children are intolerant to milk and, if so, it should be excluded from their diet and calcium obtained from green leafy vegetables. Processed food of any kind, including crisps, sweets and fizzy drinks, should be excluded or restricted to special occasions only. Food intolerances are common and may need to be investigated. The most common culprits are dairy, wheat, gluten, soya and sugar.

These children are commonly deficient in essential fatty acids, which are essential for brain development, but can be difficult to obtain from the diet. A good quality Fish-Oil supplement is recommended (vegetarian sources include Linseed or Borage oil), But be aware that many children's preparations contain Aspartame (or other artificial sweeteners/flavourings) or sugar, which have also been suggested to cause hyperactivity, so read the label carefully when buying.

For healthy motor and cognitive development, children need regular exercise, ideally on a daily basis. Computer time should be restricted to that essential to study and children should be encouraged to run, laugh, play and interact with other children as much as time permits.

In summary, chiropractic is not the cure for Learning Disorders; however for many children it can make a significant difference to their quality of life and for some, total resolution of symptoms. For all children, a fully functioning spine, a healthy diet and an active lifestyle will promote neurological development and optimum health.

CHAPTER 21

"The reasonable man adapts himself to the world; the unreasonable one persists in trying to adapt the world to himself. Therefore all progress depends on the unreasonable man."

George Bernard Shaw

Backpacks are Cool for Healthy Kids

By Paul McCrossin

School children these days appear to be under greater demands than in the past. With the advent of new technology, habits have changed and the rising levels of childhood obesity would suggest that children have become less active. We all understand that a reduction in physical activity can have negative consequences for children's health; however the wrong type of activity can also have negative effects. A great way to promote physical activity is to encourage children to walk to school, which means carrying schoolbags. If you take a look around you on the school run you will see children walking to and from school with all number of bags. Increasingly, smaller children seem to be wearing backpacks, but teenagers less so, where fashion seems to prevail over function. Using a backpack incorrectly can cause pain in childhood and may contribute to future spinal problems, just as not using one can.

So let us explore what to watch out for and how your child can best use a backpack. We generally do not associate back pain with children and, as is the case with many symptoms or illnesses, we often have the attitude that "they are kids; they will get over it and bounce back", which they generally do. So, do children get back pain? They certainly do; however it is rarely chronic, usually acute or short term in nature. Severe back pain in a child can be a cause for concern of course as the likelihood that it may be related to a pathological process (such as infection or malignancy) is more likely, although still rare in the greater context. Still, as with adults, in most cases it will be mechanical.

A study by Professor Dr Shelly Goodgold Sc.D., P.T., a physical therapist at Simmons School of Health Sciences in Boston, found that 55% of the 345 children in the study regularly carried more than the recommended 15% of their body weight in their school backpacks. A third of the students in the study reported back pain. The age range was from grades 5–8 and it was noted that the younger children carried proportionally more weight as a percentage of their body weight than the older children, due to their smaller size.[1]

It is thought that a backpack with increased weight alters the child's posture and distorts the curves of the spine. This can result in altered function, muscle fatigue and pain. The child may develop a forward head posture which is a postural distortion commonly seen in chiropractic practice with adults. A pilot study by W Chansirinukor from the School of Health Sciences, University of Sydney, noted that the weight of the backpack and the duration worn affected forward head posture. This study, while only on a small group of thirteen, suggested that altered posture was observed at percentage body weights less than 15% so even this may be too heavy. Further research into the effects of varying loads on the posture is warranted.[2]

The way a bag is carried can change walking patterns as well as altering standing postures. Carrying a bag on one shoulder, whether a backpack or sports bag, promotes a lateral bend in the spine, where using two straps (that is one over each shoulder) does not. Carrying a backpack does, however, result in a greater forward lean of the head and body in comparison to single-strapped bags.[3]

These postures, if repeated frequently (as they are over the school life of a child) may lead to spinal injury and symptoms. Generally, unless symptoms develop, the posture and bag-carrying techniques are not addressed. When symptoms do present, they may initially be mild and generalised in the back, neck and shoulders and may be dismissed or not noted, particularly in the younger population.

In a sample of 3498 students between eleven and fifteen years of age it was found that there was a high incidence of back pain with a high degree of self-reported severity and chronicity. It was found that, when controlling for some of the variables, weight as a percentage of body weight was a predictive factor for back pain. The factors that were associated with pain were walking to school, method of wear, and being female.[4]

A survey conducted by the Chiropractors Association of Victoria in 2003 of 1000 school children found that 486, or almost half, carried more than 10% of their body weight in their backpack. Many had significant back pain and they attributed it to their backpacks.

A chiropractic viewpoint is that the structure and function of the spine and how it relates to the function of the nervous system and, by implication, general health is most important.[5] A symptom can be viewed as a message or signal to alert the individual that the body is under a stress of some sort; thus it is a healthy response, not something to be ignored or blocked in most cases. This is where prevention can play a role in addressing the posture before the onset of symptoms. While wearing a backpack on two shoulders will reduce lateral bending, if it is too heavy it will promote forward head posture and leaning, which may also lead to future symptoms.

Contrasting approaches can be taken which are both valid:

1. Reduce the weight in the bag and pack it more efficiently.

2. Improve the ability of the body to handle the load.

A combination of the two is an effective approach: reduce the load on the body and improve the spinal function to allow the body to cope more effectively. A chiropractor can help on both counts, firstly by giving advice and secondly by improving the spinal function where necessary. Bad habits can physically put stress on the spine which can affect the joints and mobility resulting in irritating input into the nervous system and compensation in other areas. The area of dysfunction in the spine with associated neural changes is known in chiropractic as a subluxation, and is what a chiropractor will look for in an examination. We know that as children get older they grow and become bigger and stronger while, proportionally, the amount of weight in their bags reduces compared to their body weight. Thus it is important to make sure that younger children in particular are using a backpack and using it properly.

The Chiropractors Association of Victoria, Australia recommends:

- Backpacks should be no heavier than 10–15% of the child's bodyweight when packed.

- The backpack should be sturdy and appropriately sized – no wider than the child's chest.

- Putting comfort and fit at the top of the priority list, rather than good looks.

- Choosing a pack with broad, padded shoulder straps.

- Using both shoulder straps – never sling the pack over one shoulder.

- Using the waist straps attached – they're there for a very good reason.

- Not wearing the backpack any lower than the hollow of the lower back

- Not overloading the backpack – use school lockers and plan homework well in advance.

- Placing all heavy items at the base of the pack, close to the spine.

- Using compression straps and also using the inner pockets rather than the outermost pockets, to keep the load close to the spine.

(The Chiropractors Association of Australia, in conjunction with Marathon School Supplies, has developed a Chiropak® which is available in Australia and the UK; they also have a Physiopak endorsed by the Australian Physiotherapy Association. The Chiropractors' Association of Australia (CAA), together with Spartan and Macquarie University (NSW), joined forces to research and develop the Chiropak®. See References for contact details.)

The important features in choosing a backpack are that it is the correct size, it should not be too low or too wide, and the shoulder straps should be well-padded and wide. Compression straps on the side are also useful to stabilise the contents, as well as a waist strap to take the load on the hips. The waist strap should rest just on top of the waist bones and should not be too tight; with the waist strap attached there should not be significant weight on the shoulders, enabling two fingers to be inserted under the straps with the pack on. Depending on the size of the backpack it is useful to have internal compartments to separate and stabilise the load.

It can be said that what we do today can determine our health for tomorrow. So while encouraging our children to exercise and walk to school, it is important to make sure they get the most benefit possible by wearing their properly fitted and, of course, trendy backpack!

CHAPTER 22

"Having Down syndrome means nothing to me, I'm special like everyone else. I do not let people judge me for having Down syndrome. The important thing is how I feel about myself. On the inside I feel beautiful."

Edward Barbarnell (31 years)

There is Hope for Hopeless Causes

By Carolyn Minster

When our daughter, Perri, was born nine years ago, it was a bit of a surprise to discover that she had Down syndrome (understatement is one of my strong suits). Being a chiropractor who is also married to a chiropractor, I knew that she needed quality chiropractic care from someone who had not just received this news about their newborn daughter. So we approached a colleague, explaining to him that our new daughter had Down syndrome. His response was, "Well, I can't fix that." Well, we knew that. What we wanted for our daughter was the same thing that we wanted for all our children: a fully functioning nervous system which would give her the best go at her life.

Our colleague's response got me to thinking about how people have different ideas about what constitutes a quality life. It made me think that some people out there see health in a very black and white way. Either you are healthy (i.e. whole in a physical and mental way), or you are relegated to the hopeless cause basket. It also got me to wondering about how health professionals view those who are not whole. I have met some who look at my daughter's condition and attempt to treat that, instead of looking at her and seeing that she is like every other child in need of some assistance with her health. Fortunately, I have also met others who are outstanding at seeing my daughter as a unique individual and have supported her health and wellbeing at various crucial stages in her life. This includes some medicos as well as a number of fantastic chiropractors who have kept her nervous system functioning at its optimum.

My daughter has been a very busy girl for her short nine years of life. One of the reasons for this is that the medical profession recognises the importance of early intervention for people with intellectual disabilities and acknowledges that those with congenital defects have an equal right to access vital medical care. Her early intervention was aimed at exercising her brain to maximise her potential. This is tacit acknowledgment that these children are behind the eight ball to start with and that any assistance at this early stage is worth a lot more than therapy later. I see that chiropractic does exactly the same thing for her nervous system: it ensures there is no interference to the nerve supply so that her body and brain can function at their optimum level. Early intervention for your nervous system – why wait for the problem to get bad enough to require care? Why wait for the symptom?

Because of Perri's congenital condition, she has the most exquisitely delicate ear canals, the most robust system for producing mucous, and an immune system that likes to take long vacations. All of this means she is, by definition, prone to ear infections. I could wait for the ear infections to start, see how bad they get and then embark on some chiropractic care. In the meantime, her hearing has diminished, she can't hear instructions, can't learn properly or concentrate, and then the behaviour problems set in. I vote for early intervention which equals decreased ear infections (or, if you're like my daughter, no ear infections!!) and decreased disruption to learning. It's hard enough to learn when you have an intellectual disability, you really don't need a hearing defect as well.

Some very encouraging studies have shown that chiropractic adjustments are great for decreasing the incidence of ear infections in young children. That certainly has been my experience in practice. (See Matt Doyle's chapter.) I have had the good fortune of adjusting a number of children with Down syndrome who subsequently have less ear infections, blocked tear ducts, snotty noses and respiratory infections. This means that they are less likely to breathe with their mouth open and their tongue poking out, which, in turn, results in better muscle tone around the mouth area, meaning that it is easier to speak in a way that people can understand them. The best speech therapy – provided by a chiropractor!

"I can get a lot of money if I sell my extra chromosome on eBay. I don't need it anymore." Graham Sheldon (23 years)

Over the past few years I have had the pleasure of meeting some wonderful parents who are on similar journeys to us with their children. They don't all have Down syndrome but they do all have varying degrees of difficulty in their lives. Universally, they can do with all the extra help they can get. Our Federal government has acknowledged this in one particular example by outlaying extra funding for children with autism. This condition is undergoing an enormous increase in incidence and can put children and families under enormous stress. A lot of the children I have met in this situation have great difficulty communicating even their most basic needs. I often wonder what it would be like to need a drink of water or to go to the toilet and not be able to tell someone. What would it be like to have a headache or a stomach ache and not know how to communicate that? I think I'd be pretty cranky and there might be some people around me who would label my behaviour as difficult or inappropriate to the situation.

When parents ask me if chiropractic would be useful for their child who is on the autistic spectrum, I always keep those thoughts in mind. I'm pretty sure I don't hold the cure for autism (Oh if only!!) but I do know that chiropractic is good for these children's nervous systems. I see children who find it easier to sleep at night, who can concentrate better at school and who are just a little bit calmer and easier to spend time with. I don't care that it produces some unique situations in our clinic – that's our challenge not theirs. As a parent of a child with a disability, I know how important it is to know that you are not judged by your child's behaviour – thank goodness!! (We moved our door handles higher, only to have those crafty little children grow taller.) The rewards far outweigh the challenges and the biggest reward I get often comes from one word. When a child gets off my adjusting table and says, "Better", my day has been made a lot brighter. I guess that one word encapsulates what chiropractic aims to do. It makes life better.

Perri has a great gift for grabbing life with both hands and enjoying every bit of it. She really does dance like no one is watching, sings like no one is listening and is the absolute supreme master of loving like she's never been hurt.

As predicted by that colleague so long ago, chiropractic didn't fix my daughter's Down syndrome. What it did do was improve her life immeasurably. Her regular chiropractic adjustments allow her nervous system to work the best it can so her body and mind can go about the business of living.

CHAPTER 23

"Teaching our children to be well through our behaviours and actions today leads to a healthier world tomorrow."

Author unknown

A New Way of Looking at Kids Ear Infections

By Matthew Doyle

Your one-year-old wakes you up early in the morning, crying and grabbing her ear, which seems a lot redder than usual – it looks and sounds like an ear infection. You've seen this several times before in your two-and-a-half-year-old son, and remember the multiple episodes and the doses of antibiotics you gave him. A friend mentions she took her child with a similar problem to a chiropractor, which helped a lot – so you look into it.

Ear infections are one of early childhood's common immune system challenges and the profession of chiropractic is full of amazing examples of the benefit of chiropractic care when this challenge hits. There is a growing body of published evidence[1–11] to support these clinical experiences.

Chiropractors have been taking care of children since the early days of Chiropractic, which began in 1895.[12] Never at any stage of development does a body go through so much growth and change as from an infant to an adult. Possibly the most significant period of neurological development occurs in the first few years of life. This is where the primary goal of the chiropractor is to assist the child to be as healthy as possible through a healthy spine, a nervous system as free from interference as possible and healthy lifestyle choices.

The medical term for the common ear infection is 'otitis media' (OM). *Mosby's Medical, Nursing, and Allied Health Dictionary 6th Edition* defines it as: "Inflammation or infection of the middle ear". Children suffering from otitis media are amongst the most common visitors to the paediatrician.[8] It is one of the most prevalent childhood conditions, with 62% of children having an episode by age one and this rises to approximately 84% by age three.[13] The more chronic form, called "otitis media with effusion" (OME), is commonly known as "glue ear" – where the middle ear has a build-up of fluid in it without acute inflammation in and around the external ear.

There are a number of signs to look for, which include the five cardinal signs of inflammation: heat, swelling, pain, redness, and loss of function (hearing). The different visible areas of the ear – the pinna of the ear (the large outer cartilaginous part that sticks out), the external canal, and the bony area behind the ear – may show redness. There may be some fluid coming from the ear. The child may have signs similar to a cold or flu, such as a runny nose or an increased body temperature. They may be grabbing at their ear, complain of a sense of fullness in the ear, and be more irritable, and all this may affect their sleep. When your health care provider looks inside your child's ear, there may be a bulging of the ear drum, changes in the light reflecting back from the otoscope, or evidence of increased fluid in the middle ear.

With all this going on, it's important for you as a parent to know what options you have to help your child. Steps such as dietary improvement and eliminating allergens are simple changes you can make at home straight away. The most common culprits that may be responsible include dairy and wheat products (including gluten and yeast), nuts, shellfish, refined sugar and eggs.[14]

The medical approach to OM has generally been reliant on drugs and surgery. These are the two frontline invasive treatment options; however, significant questions have been raised in the OM literature about the rate of antibiotic prescription and the usage of tympanostomies (surgical incision of the ear drum, usually with a tube [grommet] inserted).

There are a number of concerns with the usage of antibiotics as a primary treatment for OM.[15] These include: a significant number of cases are not of bacterial origin and therefore may not respond to antibiotics; the detrimental effect of widespread antibiotic usage leading to proliferation of antibiotic-resistant bacteria; side-effects potentially linked to antibiotic usage such as increased bowel symptoms[16] and an increased risk of asthma[27]; a large body of research which does not support their effectiveness for the condition[17]; and the questioning of the general basis for which antibiotics were prescribed – which is noted to be more likely if the clinician thought the parents wanted a prescription.[18]

The most recent guidelines from the USA (2004) indicate a change of thought processes behind the treatment of OM, with a period of watchful waiting being recommended in the more common less severe cases.[19]

The surgical option is tympanostomy, and when performed is usually for the more chronic OME. A recent review by a world leader in evidence-based health care, the *Cochrane Collaboration* (current to 2010), made several important distinctions regarding this operation. They noted only short term beneficial effects in terms of the child's hearing and found most tubes came out over time, potential adverse affects on the ear drum existed, and they did not help with speech and language development, so their recommendation for most children with OME was a "watchful waiting" strategy.[20]

Chiropractic care has the potential to offer much in the health of children. It is reassuring to know that recent research has investigated and supports the safety of chiropractic care for children.[21-24] *The Journal of Alternative and Complementary Medicine* in 2007 published a systematic review which included their conclusion that the "evidence was promising for the potential benefit of manual procedure for children with otitis media".[25]

The primary theory chiropractic works on is the effect of a subluxation complex[26] on the body's ability to adapt to its environment. The major component is typically a lack of normal movement in a joint, with its concurrent effect on the local neurological signalling. From infancy through childhood, the bones of both spine and skull are not fully formed which allows greater potential for a disruption to normal function. This is particularly so when considering any traumas – caesarean section, assisted delivery such as forceps or Vontuse extraction, and the multitude of knocks and falls that come along with being a kid.

If a child has a subluxation complex, especially of the upper neck region, they may be more likely to have an ear infection for a number of reasons. The nerves from the upper part of your neck control the muscle that opens the Eustachian tube, the tube between your middle ear and the back of your throat – the one that "pops" when you yawn, or in a plane. This tube drains fluid from the middle ear, so interference to it may cause blockage.[11] The lack of normal movement may increase the firing of signals from muscles around the top of the neck, and this may affect reflex central nervous system activity to nerves going to that area, which affects the mucosa of the Eustachian tube.[5] The result may be more mucous in the tube – more mucous, more congestion, and a better environment for bacteria and viruses to grow. One of the ways your body removes unwanted guests such as these is through white blood cells. The body produces lots of them to fight off an infection, and has to drain these away to clear the area. To do this, your body needs good movement to stimulate the flow of the lymphatic system, which is restricted when there is a problem with the normal function and movement of your neck.[1]

As Dr Hawk D.C. Ph.D and co-authors concluded[25], the evidence is promising for the potential benefit of manual procedures on children with ear infections. The chiropractic adjustment to assist correcting areas of subluxation is a natural way to help the problems that appear to be involved commonly in ear infections. It improves neck joint movement, releases the tension from the muscles, allows the lymphatic system and Eustachian tube to drain the area efficiently, and gives your child's nervous system a helping hand to function as free from interference as possible. Chiropractic care helps your child's body express a greater state of health, which should assist their body to naturally improve or resolve the ear infection.

This is what I told the worried mum who brought her one-year-old daughter to me with a three-month history of constant ear infection flare ups. She'd had a tough introduction to the world: born at 36 weeks via C-section, she was the second child her mother was supposed to not be able to have. She had been hospitalised previously, surviving on a drip, with one of those bouts of ear infections. She'd been through three courses of antibiotics, surviving an allergy to the initial one. Her mum said she was generally "a quite poorly baby, but happy". She was hoping not to have to use the next course of antibiotics she had waiting. In this little one's case, her ear was inflamed, obviously sensitive, had fluid evident in the ear canal, and had not slept well the previous night. Following a thorough assessment (a discussion of the findings, risks and benefits), and Mum's ok to go ahead, I adjusted the subluxation complexes in her upper neck, and gave her mother the advice of 'watchful waiting' for any signs of deterioration and discomfort. When she attended the clinic the following day, she appeared almost a different child. She happily puttered around the room (having only just started walking) and when I examined her, she showed no sign of fluid in the canal, no discomfort with the ear, very little redness, and was reported to have slept through the night. It was the quickest change in those signs her mother had seen in any episode of ear infections she'd had. A further series of gentle adjustments to her spine were required over the next two weeks, with which she co-operated very well. She was put on a 'well child' check-up schedule over the next three months. In this time she had one mild flare up, which settled within 24 hours of an adjustment to her neck. It has been reported in the literature[1] that children who have had chiropractic care and had multiple ear infections tend to respond quicker and return to a less symptomatic state when chiropractic care has been part of their regular health care. Her mum had not had to give her the antibiotic, and was very grateful to have been able to help her daughter naturally.

A healthy, happy ending – with chiropractic, the natural option.

CHAPTER 24

"You can't learn less."

Buckminster Fuller

Happy Hormones, Happy Woman, Happy Life

By Tracy Kennedy-Shanks

Women's Health – a "bland" term for potentially challenging problems. Do you ever wish you could go out and buy a red sports car, grow your hair long, and get a tattoo? Men do – they get off easy with their mid-life crisis. Historically, women have suffered in silence.

Is this you? Bitchy, snippy and grumpy! Nobody can do anything right. Do you cry at the commercials on TV, get depressed, and can't handle the kids? Do you get the "usual" monthly backache with your period or that "normal" monthly migraine? Does your skin break out with acne even though you are over 40? Are you bloated, on top of the weight you have gained? Do you have sore breasts and your bra is un-comfortable? Do you keep a set of fat clothes for that time of the month? Are your children in trouble but can't work out why when they did the same thing yesterday and you didn't even blink. Are you tired all the time? Do you want to stay in bed or on the couch all day but you know you have to get yourself up and going, and then keep going. Does your partner make tracks to the shed when you're in "that" mood again?

How nice would it be to wake up and feel exactly the same each day? Men do ...

So, let's focus on what is different. Brain and ovaries! Okay, let's not get into the difference between the male and female brain as it is beyond the scope of this topic; let's stick to the plumbing.

In an ideal world, females develop at puberty (average age 12), go through about 40 years of menstruation (man, that is a lot of feminine products!) and then go through menopause. No dramas! Right?

The start of menstruation in teenage girls should be a smooth transition with hormone changes eventuating in regular and painless cycles. Often this experience is less than ideal. Early or late onset of puberty is not normal, neither is period pain, acne, or an evil attitude in the young woman.

In simple terms, in an ideal situation the nerve supply (brain) sends messages to the body (ovaries) through the complex network of nerves both in and out of the spinal cord. Hormones also deliver messages. The pituitary, thyroid and adrenal glands and the ovaries can all read hormone messages. The ovaries receive the incoming messages from both nerves and hormones and then produce the correct ovary hormones at the correct times. The monthly cycle goes up and down (but your moods don't). All is well in the world!

But what about when things go wrong – when there is interference to the normal process?

In less than optimum circumstances, one of the medical options is to use chemical contraception (the pill, injection or implant) to regulate the cycle. The idea is to introduce hormones at specific times of the month to tell the body what to do. The pill often comes in a blister pack with numbered days to introduce different hormones for different days of the cycle. There is often a "white" section, usually sugar tablets that is the rest time from the hormones. The process is designed to make life easy and the hormones in the pill are different strengths to trick the body and brain into a different pattern. Sometimes skipping the white or sugar pills avoids having a period all together. The "implant or injection" method of contraception is usually a constant hormone released into the body from under the skin. The down side of introducing chemicals and hormones is that all medications have side effects. For the pill, some of the serious side effects would be: sudden breathlessness, sudden and severe pain in the chest, sudden loss of vision or double vision, severe pain in a calf, or jaundice. The more common side effects might be: weight gain, headaches, loss of libido, breast tenderness, mood changes, nausea, and spotting between periods. Refer to a chemist for the full list of warnings.

The chiropractic approach and theory – Get checked and get adjusted! If the nerves from the brain send the correct messages at the correct time to the body, then the hormones work at optimal levels to allow the body to regulate itself from the inside out for the best health outcomes.

What I often hear in my office is – "Can you check my daughter and adjust her attitude?"

So how does this happen?

Imagine the nerve supply is like electricity (it actually is). We have electricity in our house; it comes in from the main power grid along high voltage wires and goes into each house on the street. Once the power is at the house it goes through a fuse box and into different circuits that then go to different areas. In your house, the different circuits have lights, power points, air conditioners and hot water systems. Switches and remote controls turn the electricity on and off.

This is like the nerve supply (electricity) of the body. The brain is the main power source that sends messages to the body and there are circuits and pathways (the wiring, switches and lights in the room) it uses to get the messages to different areas. These messages come and go along nerves, in and out of the spinal cord.

The brain turns the nerves on and off to regulate the different pathways to make the body do different things. It is the same idea as a light switch but lights and appliances can be controlled by remotes as well. The hormone messages are like remote controls. Remote controls are made with specific frequencies for certain appliances. The remote for the TV will not operate the air conditioning or the garage door. When the right remote sends the message directly to the appliance, it works effectively. The same is true with hormones: the message of the hormone is directed at specific tissues in the body, like the ovaries.

When the nervous system is working well, it is like the electricity working in the house. When things go wrong in the body, it is like the power has gone off in the house and the appliances are all on the blink. The clocks flash, the light bulbs blow, the computer freezes, the breaker switches and safety switches trip and the whole thing needs resetting. Sometimes the problems are more isolated, e.g. where a light bulb has blown. The switch is on the wall and the light is on the ceiling in the centre of the room. When there is no light we flick the switch on and off. Unfortunately, until you replace the bulb, the power will not be restored to the light. This is like nerves going to the ovaries – sometimes the switches and remotes don't turn on and off when they are designed to, then the ovaries don't send and receive the right messages and as a result the monthly cycle can be irregular. This is when the problems and symptoms become noticeable.

The second phase of the woman's hormone cycles are the childbearing years. Periods should be non-eventful with 28 days average between cycles and a regular flow for a few days. The first half of the monthly cycle is where the body builds up the hormones to support a pregnancy and the second half of the cycle is where the body decides it is not pregnant so the lining of the uterus is sloughed off ready for the next cycle. If the woman falls pregnant, in the second half of the cycle the hormones take a different direction to maintain a viable pregnancy. One of the big challenges during this stage of life is infertility. This can be a very turbulent and emotionally challenging problem for couples. The periods might be irregular or the hormones may not be triggering the right events in the woman's body at the right times. There are many combinations of challenges that may contribute to infertility in the average couple.

Imagine baking a special cake – you have to follow the recipe and have all the right ingredients combined at the right time in the right way for a perfect result. The same is true with a successful pregnancy. The body needs exactly the right conditions for fertilisation and implantation. The developing embryo follows a specific development sequence like a complicated recipe and the baby needs time to develop, like cooking a cake.

Treatment of infertility from the medical options are: chemical hormone control, follicle-stimulating drugs and complicated IVF treatments. These treatments may have significant side effects but often women in these situations feel there are no other options and they are prepared to take the risks. Hormones from IVF can create very emotionally charged feelings in an already fragile situation.

The chiropractic approach and theory: get checked and get adjusted. Ideally the body will balance the hormones from the inside out for the optimum outcome: an ideal perfectly planned, event-free pregnancy with a straightforward and trauma-free birth for both mum and bub.

What I often hear is, "I had no idea chiropractic could help me with pregnancy."

The third phase of hormone changes is menopause, at the average age of 52 (in Australia). In an ideal world, periods just stop, end of story! But often the very word "menopause" will conjure up frightening thoughts for anyone who has heard about the challenges of "change of life".

Some of the major symptoms are hot flashes/flushes, night sweats and feeling clammy, and difficulty sleeping. Emotional turbulence can include irritability, anxiety, apprehension, sudden tears, confusion, disorientation, and mood swings and depression. If that is not enough then add challenges with mental confusion, memory lapses, and fatigue. The thought of laughing makes you cross your legs and think of wearing nappies, horrific, but so is the idea of a sneeze, due to the incontinence. Loss of libido, dry vagina, facial hair, weight gain and osteoporosis are all potentially things to look forward to, and where from there?

The Medical option: take HRT drugs and hope you are not in the percentage for increased risk of cancer or heart disease as a result of the introduced hormones.

Can chiropractic help? Well if the nerve supply and hormone messages are not getting to the right place at the right time then maybe that is contributing to the symptoms. Get checked and get adjusted!

What I often hear is: "I have problems with hot flushes and can't sleep at night; can you help me?"

The chiropractic approach and theory: Get adjusted! Let the nerves flow from the brain to the spinal cord to the peripheral and autonomic nervous system so the body works from the inside out. When you adjust the nervous system and remove the interference to the pathways, the body is able to work optimally to keep everything working as nature intended and let it heal from within.

Case studies

Sharon came to see me; she has two children and is happy. She had come to the office to see if we could help with her migraines. She was improving and when we did a progress assessment of her case she asked me about her periods. Since having her children they had never really been normal and she had gone months in between cycles. She mentioned this because since starting chiropractic care, her cycle had been painless and regular for the previous few months. She asked if this could be a result of the care she had been receiving.

Judy, who had been married for years and had no children, had started chiropractic care and never mentioned anything about her desire to have children – she had been coming to the office for a back injury she sustained at work. The medical profession had done all the tests and told her and her husband that without IVF there would be no chance of getting pregnant. Now, after chiropractic care, they have three little girls and another on the way, with no IVF.

Margaret came into my office and said she had typical headaches and had done for years. She was in her late 50s, had a grown family of four, and a low-stress lifestyle. Sometimes these headaches turned into migraines lasting a few days. This had been happening less often lately, but used to be a regular occurrence in conjunction with her periods.

After a few months under chiropractic care, she reported freedom from the headaches and asked me if she should stop taking the HRT she was on and was now curious about the antidepressants prescribed at the same time. I asked her to tell me more about the reasons she started to take the medication and why she was seeking my opinion. She told me she had been taking HRT for over eight years for symptoms of menopause as she had been having headaches. Now that she was no longer having headaches, she had become concerned about the potential side effects of the HRT. She also wondered why the HRT had not stopped the headaches in eight years but after a few months of chiropractic care she was doing better. She figured the HRT had nothing to do with the change of headaches or it would have "worked" before now. I explained that the chiropractic care was to adjust the body to self-regulate and perhaps her nervous system was now more able to do that.

The human body is amazing, and will function at optimum levels given no interference.

CHAPTER 25

> *"Lance understands that chiropractic care is comprehensive by nature ... It looks at the body as an integrated whole. And for athletes, it's not just an insurance policy for right now, but it's a plan for a long, successful career."*
>
> Dr Jeff Spencer
> (Lance Armstrong's chiropractor during
> his first 7 Tour de France wins)

The Winning Edge

By Ed Groenhart

C hiropractic care has at its core the pursuit of 100% health and body function, rather than merely symptom suppression. This is also at the root of sport: the pursuit of 100% performance and continuing improvement.

Sportspeople are looking for 100% performance and continuing improvement, and chiropractic care has at *its* core the pursuit of 100% health and body function. Combining the two can certainly give the sportsperson a competitive edge.

Chiropractic is neurologically-based, focusing on all messages in the body, not just pain signals coming from a part of the body that has been significantly injured. (Pain signals from an injured tissue work on an "all-or-nothing" basis – the nerve only sends messages once trauma to a tissue in the body is significant enough to report; below this level, nothing is reported back to the brain, so nothing is "felt" by that person). Chiropractic is rather more interested in the body healing correctly in response to measured stresses applied, just as training is, in order to stimulate the body into responding positively. Ultimately, sportspeople don't want to wait for symptoms to appear. Symptoms mean time taken away from achieving and excelling in their chosen field of competition. Chiropractors don't want to wait for symptoms either, because they want a fully aligned body that can perform at 100%. Chiropractors and athletes also recognise the damage to body and mind that regular use of drugs (for avoiding disease and injury) can do, as opposed to the use of natural approaches.

Chiropractors' approach to sportspeople is really no different to their approach to anyone else: the pursuit of 100% health and continuous improvement. This is simply because everyone, whether an 86-year-old grandmother or a 19-year-old international footballer, deserves 100% health. However, the environments these people put their bodies into are entirely different, as we will see below.

So we've established that there is a core link between the foundations of sport and chiropractic: both recognise the importance of prevention being better than cure. In order to understand how we aim to prevent injuries, we have to understand what causes may lead to them. This is a study known as epidemiology. Epidemiology of injury depends on the type of sport. A 2004 study by the New Zealand Rugby Union Federation revealed that, among other things, injury is related to:

- level of competition
- sport type and position played
- time of season
- pressure to return to play

Most of the above aspects have to be taken into consideration, along with the individual health profile. This involves both the athlete and his coaches, and members of the healthcare team. Even in single-competitor sports, at an elite level the team approach is seen to be the best approach with regard to injury treatment and prevention.

At the most basic club level, a chiropractor will be working with perhaps a physiotherapist, a massage therapist and a trainer. As such, a chiropractor is often initially left with injured athletes who have not responded to conventional medical approaches. My first serious experience of sports chiropractic at a professional level was with a promising young footballer who came to my office with a persistent groin injury. Work included chiropractic adjustment, specific stretching and functional testing. Once the appropriate care had been administered and follow-up care had been provided by other members of the healthcare team, the player was back in the team, fitter and stronger than before. Noting the changes, more and more players were soon coming in for a "tune-up" *prior* to matches. Why? Because it is just as likely that changes to body function and spinal alignment can happen during training as in competition.

Indeed, increased stresses and strains of sports training and competition often lead to adaptation that the body has to make in order to continue (see any local body-building gym to see what I mean!) These increased stresses and strains lead to postural change, which necessarily means that spinal alignment and function have altered, followed often by secondary compensation in other parts of the body as more whole-body changes occur. If you're wondering what I mean, ask yourself, why does one knee always play up rather than both when they're both the same age? It's all down to relative levels of stress and strain. This is most obvious in racket sports like tennis, but can also be seen in other sports, especially if the athlete has had to compensate for an injury at some point.

Chiropractic aims to break this cycle of stress-induced adaptation and compensation by balancing posture, spine and, theoretically, the function of the Central Nervous System (CNS), even before symptoms alert the athlete to injury as a result of this stress. We can even apply this to "unavoidable" traumatic injuries that occur most often in contact sports: the body will often compensate to allow that person to continue to function, but such changes will rarely revert to normal once the primary injury has healed without help in the form of therapeutic intervention and proper rehabilitation and conditioning.

So, in theory, the chiropractic approach aims to reduce the accumulation of injury and exertion-induced changes that lead to breakdown of the body and lost performance. This applies as much to sports where the peak of physical performance is often only around five years long, such as sprint events, as to sports where season's best is more important than personal best, such as Masters athletics, where athletes over 35 years of age are less concerned with all-time achievements but have more emphasis on seasonal and "one-off" achievements in competition.

In modern society, sport is becoming more than just competition between teams and individuals; it's showbiz, with sportspeople cast as celebrity role models. The role model factor of professional sport – how a sportsperson can influence so many people into leading a healthy life with natural, drug-free approaches at the core – is in tune with chiropractic philosophy. This is epitomised by Lance Armstrong. When Lance won his seven Tour de France races he used many natural approaches, including chiropractic with Jeff Spencer, and beat many competitors who were later found to be using drugs illegal in their sport. A ringing endorsement, if ever one was needed, for drug-free healthcare and performance enhancement!

If you're still with me, you may be asking what you as a keen sportsperson can do now to make the most of your talent and reach your sports goals. You can start by following **The 5 Pillars of Health,** outlined in the "The Family Way" chapter:

1. **Correct Training and Exercise** (Consult a personal trainer or coach to refine your technique.)

2. **Hydration and Nutrition** are really important for athletes – even just checking the colour of your urine, without going into lots of physiological testing, can give you an idea of your hydration levels and give you a vital edge.

3. **Positive Mental Attitude** (PMA) and visualisation can focus your body's attention. If you're a bit sceptical about the psychological aspect of sport preparation just watch the time and effort taken by track and field sprinters pre-race to focus, and then count how many times seasoned pros talk about the importance of being "in the zone" to achieve one's best.

4. **Rest Days and Sleep** are vital to maximising your body's response to all those hours spent training. What is training for? It's to stimulate your body to respond to increased stresses and the call for a higher level of function. This can only occur after your body has had time to build and reorganise tissue.

5. **A Fully Functioning Body** completely aligned and fully controlled by its Master Control System (the central nervous system).

(Further areas that can be looked at include the quality of sleep you're getting, taking breaks from sitting at work, and following – and maintaining – a regular stretching routine.)

Training is all about perfecting the complex programs contained in the body that need to be called on with precise timing in order to carry out our sport to the highest level of physical ability. Chiropractic, in its fundamental approach, recognises that and tries to make sure the body is able to communicate with itself and balance itself in perfect harmony with the surrounding environment. This approach is not unique to chiropractic, but more and more sportspeople – like Tour de France cyclists, professional football players and international rugby teams – realise that the chiropractic approach has a key role in the athlete's health and performance support. Chiropractors realise that to "chase" symptoms alone disregards any causative or limiting factors, wastes time and, ultimately is a false economy, leading to lost performance and possibly even early retirement from sport altogether.

CHAPTER 26

"75 trillion cells, 3 billion heartbeats
600 million breaths, 30,000 days to live
500 dreams and goals, 1 lifetime
Maximise your health and your life with
chiropractic."

Author unknown

Spinal Health or Spinal Pain

By Veronica Hope

My husband and I were out for lunch last week in a village cafe close to home in Kent, and there was a man serving behind the counter that we did not recognise. I took one look at his posture and inherently knew he had neck pain and problems. Our usual waitress came over and I commented that I did not recognise the gentleman serving; she told us he was her husband who was helping out for the day. Without thinking, I said, "He looks to me as if he has got neck problems." She put her order pad down; we could see the look of surprise on her face and she said, "How do you know that?" I explained that I was a chiropractor and I described how his upper body posture showed me that he had chronic stress on his neck joints, muscles and likely his nerve system, and over time the human body has little choice but to give us pain as an indicator or signal to sort ourselves out.

So what could I see? He didn't look like the hunchback of Notre Dame and to the average person I'm sure he looked perfectly normal. Well, Mother Nature has designed our spine in a way that will ideally cope with the forces of gravity over the years and this alignment is when the head is located over the shoulders and we have a C-shaped neck curvature. You know when your mum used to tell you to stand straight head up, shoulders back – she was right. The posture of the gentleman in the cafe was far from this. He had what I would describe as severe forward head carriage, meaning his head was sitting very significantly in front of his central shoulder area and his neck looked very straight, no curvature at all. This is a very common problem and if this posture is prolonged it can create stresses on the spinal structures that can lead to pain and symptoms.

I have been a practising chiropractor helping people with back pain and conditions related to spinal problems for over twenty years, so the information I am about to share with you comes from my personal and fundamentally practical perspective of aiding individuals and families regain and maintain their spinal and whole body health, and in that process help them deal with unwanted back pains and related symptoms.

To maximise our health potential and prevent or reduce back and neck pain symptoms, my practice experience tells me we need to look at fostering normal spinal alignment, mechanics and posture over the course of our lifetime. But what is normal, how does it work and why is our spine important to our overall health? Well, let's think about it; Mother Nature has developed an incredible system in that our spine is fundamental to our posture yet is a moveable structure that allows us such flexibility, but at the same time it is strong enough to offer protection for our spinal cord and nervous system. The nervous system itself is incredible and consists of the brain, spinal cord and nerves and is literally the super freeway of electrical signals that run throughout the body enabling our life to occur while adapting us in every moment to our environment. Our nervous system is our silent lifelong partner and should be quietly running our body through the protection and safety offered to it from the spine. For example, right now you are sitting here reading this yet at the same time your heart is beating, your lungs are breathing, your stomach is digesting, your kidneys are filtrating, your liver is detoxing, your temperature is regulating, your cells are renewing and replacing themselves plus trillions of other functions to keep you alive, and the best bit is you can't feel any of it. Your life-giving physiological functions and processes are mostly occurring below conscious awareness through the amazing ability of your nervous system sending and receiving the signals of life to every cell in your body every moment of your life. So if our spine or spinal postural balance is habitually out of alignment, as with the waiter mentioned above, it places stress not only on our mechanical spinal structures and soft tissues but on the potential function of our nervous system. Over time this can lead not only to the development of back pain and related symptoms but also to a detrimental expression of the individual's fullest health potential.

When people first come to see a chiropractor it is not usually to experience their fullest health potential, but more likely to help get rid of an unwanted pain or a back-related symptom, like neck pain, headaches, low back pain or sciatica. And usually these people have tried other interventions first, like a visit to their GP with resultant medications, or maybe to a physiotherapist where exercises were the treatment. From my experience, these people are frustrated and want answers in terms of knowing what is wrong and results in terms of doing something to solve that problem and get well as quickly as possible and then, if offered the opportunity, knowledge and care in how to stay well in the future.

My job, as I see it, is to find the underlying cause of their pain and health problem. If it is from poor spinal function and alignment and its associated issues (in chiropractic we call this condition vertebral subluxation), then a chiropractor, through the art of spinal adjustment, can likely help these people to improve spinal alignment and function and, over time, make improvements in overall postural balance and help the nervous system reintegrate itself. Many times during this process a chiropractor will offer a wellness-based health re-education process including areas such as eating well, stretching and exercise, thinking well and improving posture. This can allow space in the person's mind and life for a new perspective on why they have pain in the first place and how to change or improve their lifestyle habits, alongside directly improving spinal function with chiropractic care to potentially improve immediate and long term quality of life and health, thus moving them closer to their fullest health potential.

The first thing to understand is that pain is rarely the problem itself; more often it is the body's way of telling us there is a problem.

> *I believe pain is a signal to us, an opportunity for us to address and correct recent event/impacts or ongoing life habits that are not serving us toward our fullest health potential.*

For example: angina is pain in the left chest or shoulder area, but the underlying problem is actually heart dysfunction that has usually taken years to develop through poor or unhealthy daily eating and lifestyle habits. Sciatica is pain or neuralgia, usually down the back of one leg. Just as in angina (nothing wrong with the left shoulder), nothing is wrong with the leg but it is a referred pain from irritation on the nervous system in the lower back from spinal problems that can be recent in onset from physical injury but is more often a cumulative process from all the mileage on that part of the spine under gravity, with underlying spinal subluxation. Like heart disease this condition of subluxation is often silent for years under the surface and then one day symptoms appear seemingly out of nowhere, often without any significant cause.

I often use the metaphor of an iceberg, meaning the tip of the iceberg is usually only about ten per cent of the entire structure; it's the part we can see above the water's surface and it represents the pain and symptoms we don't want. Yet underlying the water's surface, the majority of the actual iceberg exists and this represents the causes and ultimate reasons for us having the current health crisis – accumulative mileage we have done in our body over the years, plus the actual injuries and impacts like knocks, falls, car accidents and sports injuries (macrotrauma). Add to that repetitive and stressful daily postural habits like too much sitting, incorrect work postures at computers, poor sleep postures, heavy lifting etc. (microtraumas) that have all contributed to poor adaption and spinal misalignment/subluxation. Additionally, very few of us escape from experiencing significant levels of emotional and chemical stressors over the years contributed to by our nutritional status, spiritual journey and state of mind, hydration and fitness levels. This is how health issues develop and accumulate under the surface of our conscious awareness, through consistent physiological adaptation to our life's accumulated daily habits, choices and stressors, plus the impacts and injuries incurred.

Let me give you an example with a patient's case from my office. Mr A, in his early seventies, first attended in 2007 after six years of his wife suggesting he try chiropractic care with me for deteriorating health and chronic worsening low back and shoulder pain. He also was significantly overweight, suffering diabetes and high blood pressure. He described the pain as so significant he was unable to do any exercise at all, including walking, and he was suffering from feeling progressively more depressed. Mr A was on an increasing amount of medication and felt he had tried everything, including physiotherapists, massage, and osteopaths; he had resigned himself to continued deterioration.

As a chiropractor I went to his spine to look for answers. His posture was terrible, which means his spine was subluxated, causing stress not only mechanically but to his nervous system and, in my opinion, contributing to his deteriorating health and pain. Mr A had 6 cm (2.4 inches) of forward head carriage creating significant stress on his nervous system and mechanically under gravity causing accelerated wear-and-tear degenerative change to the joints in his lower neck. He also had significant spinal misalignment and subluxation in his low back affecting his mobility, because when the joints become misaligned and dysfunctional over time, loss of motion or stiffness is a very common effect. X-rays showed severe degenerative joint changes in his low back.

So, in 2007, when Mr A came to see me for help with pain and deteriorating health, I think as a last resort, I was looking at a man with a spine, nervous system and posture that had taken literally a lifetime to develop the level of deterioration and difficulties he was experiencing. Increasing pain had been present for six years but the underlying spinal subluxation causing nerve stress, postural imbalance and degenerative changes had been present much longer, mostly silently building under the surface, like the iceberg. Mr A described a car accident 30 years previous, and a number of significant sport injuries in his twenties, coupled with the usual mileage we all go through with no supportive chiropractic care for his alignment. I started working with Mr A using spinal adjustments on a twice weekly basis over a period of three months. There was a 30% improvement in his postural head carriage, his pain was significantly reduced, he started mobility exercises and walking distances, his sleeping was dramatically improved and his state of mind was more positive and hopeful. Mr A was able to get adjusted then on a weekly basis and over a period of 18 months from starting chiropractic care he regularly swam and walked, lost two stone (12.7 kg) in weight, his diabetes and high blood pressure were under control with significantly less medication and he was enjoying his quality of life with a greater level of vitality, significantly without back and shoulder pain. His head carriage posture improved more than 70 per cent. But I would like to reiterate that the pain he came to me with in 2007 was not the problem itself; his underlying poor spinal and postural alignment, coupled with his health status, were the culprits and the pain was his body's way of communicating this. So many times a chiropractor's aim is not to get rid of pain alone but to help the person return to more normal spinal alignment function and posture, coupled with positive lifestyle change to give the body the best opportunity to heal itself. How we helped Mr A rebuild his health was not with biochemistry (drugs) but by gradually working to retrain his spinal alignment with chiropractic adjustments and gentle exercises, increasing his hydration, improving his nutrition and allowing time for the nervous system and body healing systems to reintegrate themselves in a better way. As this occurred, pain signals were no longer necessary as the body was able to heal and function more normally.

Another case is Miss R, in her early twenties, who came to me for severe neck pain and headaches, loss of energy and difficulty sleeping or working because of neck pain. The problems had started after a serious fall down stairs one month earlier. She had attended her GP and physiotherapist and was on pain medication and signed off work. The pain and dysfunction were so serious she had decided to give up her job with horses and move back home with her parents to recover. Her mum and dad were patients of mine and brought Miss R to me. I found her spinal alignment, specifically in her neck, to be very subluxated with more than 4 cm of forward head carriage and a complete reversal of the normal neck curvature. There was associated muscle spasm and headaches originating from these issues and nerve system stress. Within three weeks of adjustments, all the pain issues were resolved, she was sleeping well and her energy was returning. But it took two months in total for significant improvement in her neck posture and alignment. Many times it will take longer for mechanical and structural realignment to occur than it will for the pain to go away. The longer the underlying misalignment and postural damage has been there, as in Mr A's case, the longer that structural improvement can take. Short term problems, as in Miss R's case, can be quicker to resolve, although pain usually responds more rapidly than the actual underlying spinal alignment and nerve function.

Finally, pain can be a more complex issue than alignment alone. Recently I spent time in Australia visiting my grandfather. He is in the final stages of cancer and is mostly bedridden. His mind is still fully active and he is desperately holding onto life with every breath. He told me he was having great difficulty with low back pain and couldn't sleep at night because of the pain. I said, "Pop, if you can roll on your side I can try and help." And that's what we did. Every day I would very gently massage and adjust my dear old pop's back. I honestly didn't hold out much hope that it would help as I knew it was the spread of the cancer invading his spinal bones that was causing the pain, but I wanted to try and help him. After just a week my pop was able to sleep through the night and he told me I had "fixed his back". I cried, because I knew that I hadn't really fixed anything, but I was so grateful for the magic of human touch and the gift of chiropractic that I have been given, that I could offer my beloved pop some pain relief and better quality of life in his final days.

Just imagine how it would be if people used chiropractors not only to help get rid of pain but to actually stay healthy. My vision is that we all take care of our spinal alignment through regular chiropractic adjustments so chiropractic becomes part of our healthy lifestyle choices like eating well, exercising regularly and thinking positively. In my opinion we could avoid so much unnecessary suffering, as in Mr A's case, and we could promote and encourage a completely new level of health consciousness and understanding about the human health potential. Just imagine if we all actually gave attention to maintaining and facilitating the health of our spine, posture and nervous system over the course of our lifetime, how that could positively influence our whole body – our flexibility, vitality, and ability to stay physically active. Fundamentally, our nervous system would be clear to best communicate throughout our system to our entire body.

Give yourself and your family the opportunity to experience the gift of chiropractic.

CHAPTER 27

"The scientist knows, that in the history of ideas",
observes Michael Gaugelin in The Cosmic Clocks,
"magic always precedes science, that the intuition of
phenomena anticipates their objective knowledge."

D. Church
(P 45, *The Genie In Your Genes*)

Genetics vs Epigenetics – The Glass Box

by Maryellen Stephens

The pain in my coccyx is so intense I can barely sit, but sit I do, and the midwife hands me this gorgeous screaming pinking up baby (girl I note, as I peek down!). My first daughter, Abby, has wandered back into the room, and kneels beside me and cuddles us, eyes wider than saucers. I am laughing and smiling and crying all at once. I am beyond delighted. I find myself checking her fingers and toes, looking into her lovely little eyes as they peer up at me half open. Her milky skin, and fatty umbilical cord. And her palms – I realise that I am looking to see if she has one crease or two. And the thought almost stops me in my tracks, thinking of all the medical tests I have refused with both children, not wanting to know, not wanting to be invaded or to risk her life, simply because it wouldn't change anything for me. I wanted these children, and love them I would – purple, blind, Down syndrome or otherwise.

She is Holly.

I laughingly remember back to the days when Dad was trying to teach me Mendelian law for science class: big B and little b genetic squares. Will they have brown eyes or blue? How simple it all seemed then, and vague and impersonal. Not quite like the families I have come to know now, having children with ZFHX1B chromosome 2 region 2q22 (Mowat-Wilson), CFTR deltaF508 mutation (Cystic Fibrosis), SMN1 (Spinal Muscular Atrophy), or 22q11.2 deletion (Di George) to name a few. Suddenly the whole concept of 'autosomal dominant', 'recessive', and 'x-linked' takes on a very personal meaning.

A father, who has seen us for his low back pain, comes in with his child who just doesn't seem to be like other children. Others see pictures of kids on our walls, or their friend's cousin's niece or grandchild comes here …

Could we help? Could we do anything to help their child?

These are the people who keep me up at night, make my eyes water and my heart ache with joy, anticipation, inspiration and sadness. I want to "fix" them all, and I know I can't. And I know it really isn't about that. It's about finding who they are and what they can do in their little lifetimes. Some are so short; others are long and full. Our job/mission as chiropractors is to be part of the discovery of what that FULLness means. For those who were told that their particular syndrome meant they would never walk, and then do… for those who are told that their child will never connect meaningfully with them, and then do… for those who have only a little time to live, making it an easier time for them in any way possible.

This is what matters.

Caring for children with any genetic syndrome means walking where many fear to tread. There is very little research to support chiropractic care for these children and families; most exists as anecdotal evidence and case studies from chiropractors worldwide and parents who have seen remarkable and life-affirming changes in their children. And if there is one thing that I have learned in my heart and in my bones, it's DON'T GIVE UP ON YOUR CHILD.

DON'T GIVE UP ON YOUR CHILD.

If there is nothing else that you can do (other than LOVE THEM) in their little lifetimes, it is that one thing.

And it's a big ask.

These children change *everything* for their families. Hopes and dreams, marriages, family relationships, sibling relationships, *all of it*. There's a huge range of emotions, from rage to despair to guilt, blame, anger, and grief … and then out the other side with love and grace and gratitude. *Every family goes through it*, and all come to peace in their own time and in their own way – together or apart.

So many things strike me with each new family I meet. Mostly it's that the information they have is so coldly accurate, but limited to a medical perspective. Their child has been diagnosed and they are given a glass box full of information; medical information and glass ceilings of limited expectations. Within any given syndrome there may be an inherent variability in expression of the features. It is this, and the fact that many of these children have never had functional neurological care, that allows us the hope for positive support for the body to do what it needs to do, *and can do*, to help heal itself on whatever level. How do we know if we haven't challenged the system to see what can change? What can grow? What can evolve over time into a healthier, more vital and connected child? There are many roads to travel when you smash that glass box and allow hope to enter your heart – even if it's solely opening the door to other parents and sharing your experiences.

So where is the hope? Where does it lie? The science of epigenetics (changes in gene expression due to factors outside the DNA sequence) has opened up the minds from the "quiet" side of medicine, one that believes (as chiropractors do) in the body's innate ability to change through generations, and believes in HOPE. One of the hardest things about understanding genetics is understanding that it is beyond us. It's before us and after us. Not us – we are the expression of what is the result of the ancestral past and the potential of what could be for our future generations. Native communities speak of how one life affects the seven generations before and after. Our genes are not about who we are – they are about who our ancestors were and who our children and future generations will be. Therein lies the key to the "kingdom", so-to-speak. If you can get your head around the concept that you are not one life, that you are the result and expression of the many lives before you *and will be the foundation of the many lives that come after*, then your health and your lifestyle, and the expression of health in terms of your genes and genetics, takes on a whole new meaning.

There is still the unknown, the untapped potential of what we are capable of in terms of fullness of genetic expression, and the function and purpose of genes. Chiropractic care isn't about curing a genetic syndrome in its current form. On one hand it is about finding the path to optimal functional expression, while on the other, being part of enhancing the body's innate ability to maintain its homeostasis (the body's ability to maintain a natural "set-point" to regulate its inner environment to retain stability) and healing capacities. This, in turn, leads to strong immunity and protection of normal cellular function – the root of many generational/familial/hereditary syndromes and lifestyle diseases when this mechanism breaks down.

In chiropractic terms, this means caring for families from the pre-conceptive stage and beyond. It means doing everything we can to prepare the body on all levels for a healthy conception (mother and father), pregnancy and delivery. It means caring for a family as a whole as they grow into adulthood and beyond.

Is it possible to affect the outcome on a genetic level? Is it possible to change the genetic destiny of a family? In terms of modern science and a long view, I believe it is. Maybe not in my lifetime or one generation, but in several; the possibility exists. If your family were carriers of the gene for Huntington's Chorea, breast cancer, spinal muscular atrophy, cystic fibrosis, Down syndrome or ... what would this change for you? We are already seeing examples in the scientific literature of just these sorts of changes in animal studies. The example of the Agouti mouse, obese and diabetic for generations, suddenly becomes lean and healthy with the addition of folate, vitamin B12, betaine and choline to the mother's diet (see *The Biology of Belief*, Bruce Lipton pages 70–73); genetically identical to the mother, but with no expression of the gene that causes the illness. Consider the use of folate in pregnancy to prevent neural tube defects in newborns. No one can guarantee a perfect outcome, but wouldn't you do everything you could do anyway, regardless, to optimise the health of your future children?

What are the things that can affect cellular function? What has a direct influence on our genetic destiny that is within our grasp? Neurological dysafferentation (abnormal input into the central nervous system leading to an abnormal or inappropriate response – chiropractors call this the vertebral subluxation complex), lifestyle issues (such as nutrition, fitness, prescription and recreational drug use), and STRESS!

With generational thinking applied, the science of epigenetics gives us a new level of approach, an accessibility that was beyond our vision beforehand. We may not be able to change who we are genetically, but we can change the expression in our own lives and the lives of our future children, be it by chiropractic care, nutrition, meditation, prayer, exercise, hormonal balance, emotional clarity (our experiences and beliefs), and altering our stress patterns and lifestyles by this awareness – the being and the doing of things that create real health and communication on a cell-to-cell level.

So I invite you to smash the glass box and find the hope that exists within to inspire you to be part of creating the possible future for your children, your grandchildren, their children and all who follow.

And may it be vibrant, healthy and FULL.

CHAPTER 28

*"Natural forces within us are
the true healers of disease."*

Hippocrates

Easy Breathing Asthma

By Rob Sandford

C hiropractic doesn't treat asthma. Yet if you speak to almost any chiropractor around the world, undoubtedly they will have a success story relating to a client with asthma, breathing problems or a respiratory disorder. I am one of those chiropractors. I am also one of those clients.

I was born with a shadow on my lung. For the first four months of my life I suffered almost constant breathing problems and was plagued by a chest infection. This was accompanied by what can only be described as "explosive" digestive dysfunction! Frighteningly, the medical doctors thought I had cystic fibrosis and were testing me to confirm it.

Fortunately (for me and her) my mother had been seeing a chiropractor for some time regarding her own health problems, and a lack of childcare meant that I travelled with her. As a last act of desperation and fearing the potential diagnosis I had been given, she eventually let the chiropractor check my spine when I was four months old. Within four visits my chest was clear.

Chiropractic doesn't treat asthma or breathing problems, but it certainly changed my life.

In simple terms, asthma is a predisposition to chronic inflammation and reversible narrowing of the airways (bronchi) and lungs. There is a wide range of severity and some people with asthma only rarely experience symptoms, usually in response to triggers. Other more severe cases may have marked and debilitating airflow obstruction at all times.

Asthma exists in two states:

1. the steady-state of chronic asthma
2. the acute state of an acute asthma attack.

The symptoms are different depending on what state the sufferer is in.

Common symptoms of asthma in a steady-state include: nighttime coughing, shortness of breath with exertion but none at rest, a chronic "throat-clearing" type cough, and a tight feeling in the chest.

During acute asthma attacks (exacerbations of asthma), the smooth muscle cells in the bronchi tighten, the airways become inflamed and swollen, and breathing becomes more difficult. In extreme cases, the sufferer will be so short of breath they may lose consciousness and even die.

What is truly alarming about asthma is not only its frightening incidence rate – 7% of the US population[1], 5.2 million Britons (constituting 4.1 million GP visits per year)[2], and 300 million worldwide[3] – but also the steep increase over the last 30 years. Estimates range, but a 2006 report by Asthma UK indicated that the number of adults in the UK with asthma has increased by 400,000 since 2001.[2] An earlier study found an increase of approximately 4.3% per year from 1980 to 1996.[4] The number of children diagnosed with asthma has increased from 4% to 10% between 1964 and 1989 according to one study[5], whilst another identified a 100% increase in the same geographical region over a 15-year period from 1973 to 1988.[6] All researchers agree that the increases are due to more than a greater readiness to diagnose the condition. Clearly, asthma is an increasing and ongoing significant health concern in the UK and around the globe.

Chiropractic doesn't treat asthma; however it's also important to understand that neither does the traditional medical approach of beta-2 antagonist medications, such as Salbutimol, Ventolin or Becotide, or steroids. Even if we put aside the body of evidence which suggests that the long-term use of these medications is ineffective[7-14], it's important to appreciate that they are administered merely in an attempt to treat the symptomatic effects of asthma. This is all medicine can ever do. As such it represents sick care, not health care.

Understanding the true impact of medication on the body, the difference between sick care and health care, and the impact that chiropractic can have on an asthma sufferer, starts with the fundamental truth that health is normal.

From this understanding comes the realisation that if you're not healthy, then something is interfering with that normalcy. Often under these circumstances the body will be giving you a warning sign – a symptom. Merely removing the warning sign does nothing about the health problem, in the same manner that removing the oil light in your car does nothing to correct the oil leak.

Thus comes the distinction between sick care and health care. Sick care is the attempt to alleviate a symptom regardless of the underlying problem, i.e. removing the oil light. Medical intervention represents drugs to numb pain, artificially raise or lower performance levels, chemically relax muscles, or surgery to remove body parts. All of which will rarely directly impact the health problem itself, although they may remove the symptom. That is to say the underlying cause of the change in performance, the oil leak, is still there.

> *Sick care serves a vital function in life-saving situations, but true health care requires restoring the normal state of the body – in other words, fixing the oil leak.*

Since doctors or drugs can't heal, the only thing that the best doctors of any type can do is to remove any interferences preventing your body from expressing your normal health potential. This represents true health care.

That's why the focus of chiropractic is on your nerve system, which controls and regulates every aspect of your health and wellbeing. If controlling and regulating nerve impulses are compromised somewhere between your brain and your body (often along the spine), then restoring better brain-body communications can lead to a more normal expression of health. The fact that your headache, back pain or breathing symptom may improve in the process is as wonderful as it may be unpredictable. The alleviation of symptoms so often reported by asthma sufferers through chiropractic care is merely an expression of better nerve system control of your body.

Chiropractic doesn't treat asthma, because chiropractic doesn't treat anything. Chiropractors locate and reduce any disturbance to the nerve system resulting from misalignments of the spine. These vertebral subluxations (spinal misalignments) interfere with your ability to be fully you. Being fully you includes everything from turning, bending, walking and sleeping to breathing, fighting infection, digesting food and healing a cut.

Chiropractors correct these spinal misalignments with an adjustment that restores the integrity of your nerve system. Following the correction, your body is more likely to work as it was designed to. For some, that occurs quickly. For others, whose healing ability is limited by stress, poor nutrition, negative emotions or other factors, it occurs more slowly. Regardless, without the interference the performance of your body is enhanced and it no longer requires the warning sign. Thus the symptom will often resolve.

The vertebral subluxations occur in response to excessive trauma on the body. This trauma may take the form of physical stress such as falls, birth trauma or accidents. It could also be in the form of chemical stresses such as diet, smoking and drugs or even emotional or mental stresses. Of course your life is littered with these stresses and mostly your body will adapt and resist them, but when the resistance is overcome, damage or distortion can occur. Sometimes the damage is minor or even temporary, resulting in either no obvious symptom (although your body's performance will undoubtedly have been impacted) or a short-lived symptom. This is often characterised by repetitive episodes of symptoms or recurring problems. On other occasions the distortion may be more significant and the resultant change in body performance and health status more obvious.

My own history was of a traumatic foetal and birth experience. Due to hormone-related health problems, my mother was unaware of being pregnant until I had developed to 18 weeks. Unfortunately, during this time she had been taking strong medication, including steroids. Having reached the arbitrary cut-off point of 10 days over my due date (apparently accurately calculated despite the fact that the pregnancy was only established 18 weeks into development!) my birth was then pharmaceutically induced before either myself or my mothers' body was ready. Finally, I emerged with the cord around my neck preventing me from breathing.

It is easy to see how the resistance of my own system may have been overcome and misalignments or damage may have occurred. Evidently the resultant vertebral subluxations impacted the nerves feeding my lungs and bowel sufficiently to lower function. The symptoms I had were the result of that lowered function. Once the vertebral subluxations were removed, normal function was restored.

Unfortunately, due to the significant nature of the damage in my spine, although my normal health returned rapidly, a weakness was left in the region. When I reached puberty, breathing problems and a persistent cough returned. The GP diagnosed asthma, but I returned to the chiropractor and once again chiropractic care (along with dietary and lifestyle changes) enabled me to avoid the prescribed medication. For the remainder of my adolescence I was without symptoms or the need of this medication, and this has continued into adult life.

The area of the spine most commonly linked to asthma, as in my case, is the thoracic or mid-spine. The nerves exiting the thoracic spine feed the lungs and the bronchi. Research has confirmed a link between the mobility of the thoracic spine and lung function.[15] However, the upper neck, via its connection to the smooth muscle of the bronchi and diaphragm, has also been associated.[16,17]

Multiple studies demonstrate increases in lung function following chiropractic care.[16-21,23-25] By impacting the lungs with the chiropractic adjustment, chiropractors and their clients can anticipate a reduction in asthma symptoms, a reduced requirement for medication, and an improvement in quality of life.

The response to chiropractic care is reported to be greatest in children.[22] This may relate to the shorter duration of the spinal and nerve dysfunction, or to the increased adaptability of children. One study indicated that 92% of parents of asthmatic children who received chiropractic care considered it to be beneficial.[23]

The benefits for adults are also evident though. A 1978 study concluded that 76.5% of patients with bronchial asthma reported a benefit from chiropractic care.[19] In 2000, a study of 47 asthma cases ranging from mildly persistent to severely persistent found that symptoms not only improved dramatically under chiropractic care but improvements were also maintained. Results were based on subjective and objective reports as well as medication use. All 47 cases demonstrated significant improvement from 87–100% and all 47 reported the improvement had been maintained after two years.[26]

Chiropractic doesn't treat asthma, but the evidence that it can have a positive effect on the sufferers and the resultant symptoms is increasing. Importantly, with chiropractic care the objective is not to alleviate the symptom but rather enhance your health. With that can come a greater level of function, an enhanced healing capacity, a better lung function and less suffering from the symptoms of asthma.

As one of those helped by chiropractic care I will be forever glad that I was given the opportunity to discover chiropractic and the effect it can have on health.

CHAPTER 29

"The doctor of the future will give no medicine,
but will interest her or his patients in the care
of the human frame, in a proper diet, and in the
cause and prevention of disease."

Thomas A. Edison

Heartburn?
Relief is at Hand

By Roger Wood

Jean's Story

In August 2008, Jean was referred to me by a long-standing patient who
had experienced great benefit from chiropractic care for chronic digestive
problems. Jean (59 yrs old) was used to leading an active life but for 20 years
she had been troubled by the symptoms of Gastro-Oesophageal Reflux Disease
(GORD) and a hiatus hernia. She could recall times as a child of suffering from
bouts of acid reflux, but through the years the symptoms had worsened, and
she complained of a constant feeling of choking or needing to cough to clear
her throat. Her medical doctor felt that there may have been some damage
from the long term exposure to stomach acid, but an endoscope the previous
year had not revealed any significant complications. Jean was constantly aware
of the symptoms of GORD in the throat but particularly had trouble with

acidic and spicy foods, hot drinks, bending over forwards and sleeping with a low pillow. Jean found eating particularly difficult and frequently needed sips of water to help wash the food down. Medication offered some benefit and over the previous six years had helped by suppressing the production of stomach acid. Interestingly, she did comment on experiencing some tenderness in the mid-back.

When I examined Jean, I found significant spinal dysfunction at key levels in the neck (nerve supply to the diaphragm), the mid-back (to the stomach) and mid-lower lumbar spine (lower digestive tract). Muscle tension and tenderness was evident over the mid- back spinal levels and, not surprisingly, tenderness and increased muscular tension was evident in her diaphragm. Jean was also stuck in a classic "chest breathing" pattern.

Considering the number of years Jean had experienced symptoms of GORD and the presence of a hiatus hernia, we began chiropractic care with more of a longer plan in mind and the probability of a slow improvement. It was encouraging that the endoscope had not suggested anything of concern and our initial focus was on improving Jean's mid- back spinal dysfunction. I also gave her some breathing exercises to improve diaphragm function and to move her away from chest breathing.

We were both very happy to find that within a handful of appointments, Jean was experiencing a reduction in the need to clear her throat with a cough. We continued to focus on the relevant spinal levels of dysfunction that were also associated with the nerve supply to the stomach and diaphragm. We were soon able to use more manual adjusting techniques as the mid-back tenderness reduced. Jean was shown how to do the "diaphragm cough-reflex" herself and we continued to make good progress. Just over a month after starting chiropractic care, at our first progress examination, Jean was talking without coughing and eating without choking or using water to wash down her food! Over the next three or four months, she continued to make steady improvement and found that her eating tolerance to different foods was improving. Within only six months of care and after over 20 years of problems, Jean commented on experiencing "hardly any problems with the stomach". She was able to look forward to social lunches and dinners out with friends and family when in the past she became apprehensive about what she could order to eat or choking on the food and having to gulp water to get the food down.

In no way do I think that Jean's stomach problems have been "cured" but as long as the spinal-nerve connection and the stomach-oesophagus-diaphragm relationship remains working well, then I am sure that the next 20 years of her life with a hiatus hernia look really promising.

It is always interesting at a patient's progress examination to hear what benefits they feel they have gained from chiropractic care. A number of patients also comment on gaining additional benefits to their original complaint. Some of the most commonly mentioned additional benefits include: improved sleep, reduced or better tolerance to stress, an increased feeling of wellbeing and, frequently, an improvement in digestion.

In my experience, one of the most common digestive disorders that chiropractic patients report benefit from is heartburn (or acid reflux). Medically also referred to as Gastro-Oesophageal Reflux Disease (GORD), this is when stomach acid leaks back up the oesophagus (food pipe) causing an acidic, burning discomfort. The condition can also be exacerbated by the presence of a hiatus hernia, when part of the stomach is protruding through the diaphragm up into the chest.

The symptoms of GORD include:

- Heartburn, characterised by a burning sensation that rises from the stomach or lower chest up towards the neck.

- Regurgitation of acid into the throat or mouth that causes an unpleasant acidic, sour taste and sometimes a feeling of choking, and a cough.

The Medical Approach

Conventional medical approaches to GORD consider a number of possible causes. One of the main causes relates to a problem with the lower oesophageal sphincters (muscles) which work as a kind of gate that allows food down into the stomach but prevents stomach acid from leaking back up into the oesophagus. Other causes may include increased pressure in the stomach, the over-production of stomach acid, and the stomach taking longer than normal to dispose of stomach acid. In many cases there is no apparent reason to explain why a person has developed GORD.

Medical treatment plans for GORD are mainly aimed at drug treatment, lifestyle changes and, in some cases, surgery:

- **Medication**, which includes:

  - **Antacids** that help to neutralise the stomach acid.

  - **Alginates** that work by producing a protective "raft" that floats on the stomach contents to reduce reflux and to protect the lining of the oesophagus from the stomach acid.

  - **Proton pump inhibitors** that inhibit the secretion of gastric acid produced by the stomach.

  - **H2-receptor antagonists** that block the effects of histamine which is used by the body to produce stomach acid.

  - **Prokinetics** that may improve gastro-oesophageal sphincter function and accelerate stomach emptying.

- **Lifestyle changes,** like avoidance of excess alcohol and aggravating foods such as fats, weight reduction, smoking cessation, and raising the head of the bed.

- **Endoscopic treatment,** which can involve stitching, burning or injections administered via an endoscopic tube via the mouth.

Many people do not consider the long-term complications that can occur from heartburn. Oesophageal ulcers can form when the excessive acid produced damages the lining of the oesophagus. This can cause bleeding and pain and make swallowing difficult. Repeated damage can lead to the formation of scar tissue (oesophageal strictures) in the oesophageal lining that can narrow the food pipe and make swallowing painful and difficult. Repeated episodes of GORD can also lead to changes in the cells of the lower oesophagus, causing a condition called Barrett's Oesophagus. There is a small chance of these cells becoming cancerous.

Considering the above, it is obvious that repeated episodes of heartburn or acid reflux are not to be ignored; yet it is surprising how many patients refer to "normal heartburn". A digestive system operating at its optimum would not display the symptoms associated with GORD.

It is always beneficial to chiropractors when a patient has already had medical tests and endoscopic procedures regarding the symptoms of GORD. When considering the possible causes and complications associated with repeated and chronic heartburn/acid reflux a thorough medical assessment and examination (preferably involving endoscopic examination) is of clinical importance. However, many people are looking at more holistic, conservative approaches to managing chronic, uncomplicated digestive disorders. Because of chiropractic's conservative, holistic and drugless approach to health, many patients consult a chiropractor rather than favour the drug-based, medical approach.

Many patients are wary of known side effects and the way medications change the body's natural physiology. One wonders how often one problem may be replaced with another. Wouldn't it make more sense to try to support and help the body to re-establish the balance or homeostasis of stomach acid regulation – especially in mild to moderate, uncomplicated cases?

The Chiropractic Approach

It is important to stress that chiropractors do not "treat" GORD in a medical sense.

"Chiropractic is concerned with the diagnosis, treatment and prevention of mechanical disorders of the musculoskeletal system and the effects of these disorders on the function of the nervous system and general health." (World Federation of Chiropractic, 1999), therefore their primary aim is to locate spinal malfunction (subluxation) and re-establish optimal spinal, muscular and nervous system function at this level. Many sufferers of heartburn complain of pain between the shoulder blades and report relief following chiropractic adjustment of the mid-back. This is not a surprise when you consider the nerves at these spinal levels have links to the stomach.

An important consideration in adopting a holistic approach to optimal digestive health is a patient's lifestyle. Physical, chemical and emotional stressors affect how the body functions. It is fairly obvious that a patient's diet (chemical) is a major factor in how the body regulates stomach acid. I am in favour of a patient recording their weekly dietary habits using a Food-Mood Diary. This involves the patient recording exactly what they eat and how they feel during and after eating. The goal is to identify any dietary triggers or sensitivities related to their heartburn and often it is quite enlightening for the patient as to what they are actually eating and how the digestive system is functioning. A diet high in poor fats, processed foods, fried foods, dairy, cereals, caffeine, meat, artificial flavours, colourings, sweeteners, sugar and alcohol will not support optimal digestive function. A heavily acidic diet is obviously not beneficial.

It would be important for a person suffering from GORD to have a diet higher in alkaline foods favouring food that is whole, natural and fresh. A good supply of quality water is also vital.

Other lifestyle considerations include not smoking, being mindful of the size and timing of meals, exercise – our modern sedentary lifestyles have a lot to answer for – and dealing with emotional stress.

The Diaphragm and Hiatus Hernia

In my experience, a large number of patients with GORD symptoms have increased tension in the diaphragm. They have a tendency to switch away from diaphragm breathing to chest breathing patterns – often also found in asthmatics, patients with a chest infection, patients in longstanding stress or anxiety patterns, or following prolonged periods of coughing where the diaphragm has become stressed or fatigued. Because of the close relationship between the stomach, oesophagus and diaphragm, some chiropractors use light chiropractic techniques on the diaphragm and stomach. Optimal diaphragm tension and function is very important in re-establishing proper stomach and oesophagus function. In many cases, a specific manual chiropractic "cough-stretch-reflex" technique on the diaphragm can be of particular benefit – it "resets" the muscular tension in the diaphragm. Many patients also benefit from being able to do this technique themselves. I also give patients a breathing exercise to re-establish diaphragm breathing patterns.

Normally, the oesophagus (food pipe) enters the abdomen through a hole (the hiatus) in the diaphragm. A hiatal hernia is an anatomical abnormality in which part of the stomach protrudes upwards through the diaphragm into the chest. As the stomach lies just under the diaphragm, the function of the diaphragm can have a significant effect on the normal function of the oesophagus and stomach. When hiatal hernias produce symptoms (many do not), they frequently give the symptoms of GORD or its complications, as it can interfere with preventing acid reflux back up the oesophagus. Treatment for hiatal hernia usually follows that of the symptoms of GORD, and larger more severe hernias may require surgery.

Many chiropractors also use visceral (internal organ) techniques. One such technique places importance on the position and function of the stomach, particularly in the presence of a hiatus hernia. Often used in conjunction with the above-mentioned diaphragm release technique, the chiropractor gently but firmly places pressure onto the stomach and then gently applies a downward pressure as the patient deep breathes. In my experience, this has been highly beneficial to hiatus hernia sufferers and given quick relief in many cases.

Whilst I cannot over-emphasise the importance of a thorough medical examination and/or consultation, I hope that after reading this chapter, and in particular Jean's story, many gastric reflux suffers will look more at the drugless approach of chiropractic and what it may have to offer. This is a very exciting area of chiropractic care and it is hoped that through the years more needed research in this area paves the way for chiropractic care becoming more the conservative approach of choice than an "alternative".

CHAPTER 30

> *"Every human being is the author of his/her*
> *own health or disease."*
>
> Buddha

Why Mum was Right

By Sandy Clark

Mum always said, "Stand up straight", but to understand our posture I would like to start at the beginning. When we first start growing from two cells into billions of cells it is the differentiation of the primitive brain and spinal cord in the first six days of gestation that makes all the cells communicate with each other and play a part in each and every interaction of the whole. These cells then give rise to a network of communication for every other cell to work from. These first cells represent the foundation of all body responses and the foundation of why chiropractic care works so well for so many people. This is also the foundation of why and how we as humans can do what we do. The next group of cells to form are the ones that make up the vertebrae of the spine.

So before you are born, the nerves are controlling every part of your developing body, even the position of your spine. This brings us to your posture.

Posture is a learned system to maintain mobility, keep us upright and keep our eyes seeing with binocular vision and our ears hearing in stereo. Nearly all of our muscles are used in maintaining our posture, however the muscles closest to the spine are the most important ones that respond to and are the greatest contributors of our postural awareness via the feedback mechanism that is our nervous system.

This feedback mechanism uses the nerves that connect with and coordinate information from our whole body, i.e. from the position of our eyes, the balance centres in our ears, the position of our head and neck, the muscles and joints of our feet and even from the position of our jaw. One of the most important parts of your postural reflex system is at the brainstem. This is found at the bottom of the brain and the top of the spinal cord. It is protected by the base of the skull and the top three vertebra of the spine: Atlas (C1), Axis (C2) and C3. All the information coming from the body goes to our brainstem then to the coordination centre of our brain (the cerebellum) and then to the cortex of the brain (the top part) and back out to our body. This relay of information from body to brainstem to brain and then from brain to brainstem then back to body continuously, is the primary mechanism of all communication and comprises a large part of our reflex system.

Postural reflexes develop and are enhanced by feedback from our environment, like your feet "talking" to your brain and asking if your eyes and ears are ok etc. This whole system of feedback and brain-to-body "talking" is set in place from the moment we are born, then is enhanced, recalibrated, and relearned as we first start to crawl, sit, stand and walk. In an infant around six months old there is a postural reflex called a propping reflex that co-ordinates arm movement with body posture and corrects movement from a seated position so that they don't fall over. In fact, all of our reflexes that are present at birth have a postural component to them.

When studying chiropractic at university, after the first three years of what is, for all intents and purposes, a pre-med course, chiropractors spend two more years studying advanced neuroanatomy, neurophysiology and the spine, and further their skills in adjusting as well as continuing to further their knowledge of reflex responses to muscles and joints. Then they apply this knowledge of neurology to the relationships of organ and body function as well as body reflex systems to their knowledge of cellular metabolism, cell-to-cell communication, disease and pathology, movement, posture and life. At graduation, a chiropractor is completely versed in the assessment of an individual's health, wellness and their reflex responses to disease processes. How an individual's posture relates to their health can be seen in how they carry themselves through life – sicknesses, frailty and fitness can all be seen in our posture.

We are designed to move, to heal, to think, and all of these activities require us to interact with our environment in a specific way. If our health is being affected by something, whether it is external or internal, then it is first seen as a change in the defence and interaction systems of our body. These changes can be seen, and even measured, as sensory changes, feeling unwell and tired, or getting sick. Our body's reflex response to all of these things is a propping up of our natural abilities. Through feedback mechanisms in our body we take in the necessary information in order to heal.

How chiropractic care helps posture

These feedback mechanisms that we are talking about, when it comes to posture, I refer to as "perception".

Perception is having an awareness of elements of the environment through physical sensation. Our ability to perceive where we are in our environment and then make postural changes accordingly that allow us to adapt to this is due to perceived postural awareness. When the feedback mechanism of our body isn't working due to neurological interferences, a change in perceived postural awareness can bring about a correction to our posture leading to symptoms like vertigo or dizziness, nausea, motion sickness, foot and ankle pain, knee pain, back pain and even a decrease in life span. This has been studied in 2005 (Spine: 30(18), Sept 15, pp2024–2029) and in 2004 (J Am Geriatric Soc 52:1662–1667) showing that a forward head carriage past neutral, not only increases the severity of symptoms that a client presents with, but it also is shown to increase the mortality of these individuals with forward head carriage; i.e. the more forward the head is sitting from neutral the more likely they experience pain and have a shortened life span.

What is posture?

Our posture enables us to have free-flowing movement. It provides stability and strength in an ever-changing environment, allowing us to adapt, to change, to express our emotional state and to present ourselves to our peers. Our posture is how our nervous system presents itself to the world. In their definitive book on body language, Allan and Barbara Pease gave the world an insight into how important posture is and how your posture and your body language can tell others about your hidden emotions and truths.

Try hunching over, rolling your shoulders forward, frowning and slumping/slouching your lower back – now try and maintain this posture while you smile your biggest smile, let yourself feel open, alive and happy and take in a deep, rejuvenating breath. Were you able to maintain your slumped slouching posture? No! Your emotional state is expressed outwardly through your posture. Your inner body's life is expressed outwards in the way you carry yourself.

When I assess a client's posture and movement, I am looking at the individual's adaptation and compensation to everything they have done in their past. Chiropractors use their knowledge of reflex responses in muscles and joints and then apply this to a client's postural assessment. This tells me a lot about how they will respond to their environment in the future and I can quickly and accurately point out to the client where they are having problems with their posture and where they may be experiencing pain and why.

By the application of specific adjustments to vertebrae, extremity joints or to the cranial vault, I encourage the body to make the necessary changes to the reflex-response system that will then in turn allow the client to alter their response to their environment. This is then seen in an alteration to a client's posture, an increase in energy levels, and even as an improvement in the client's sense of wellbeing.

This mechanism of perceived postural awareness affects every aspect of our quality of life and is supported by a study of clients under chiropractic care carried out in 2001 by Network Chiropractors. When asked questions regarding their improvements in physical state, mental/emotional state, responses to stress, improvements in life enjoyment as well as in their overall quality of life, the responses reported a 76% improvement in all areas. This study was carried out with 2800 participants who reported continual improvements in all areas assessed over time and such improvements were seen from as early as three months under care and continued for those who were under care for greater than three years.

Have a chiropractor assess your posture, have your nervous system interferences corrected, enhance your feedback, improve your perceived postural awareness and start reaping the benefits of greater and greater improvements in your life enjoyment.

CHAPTER 31

"Strait is the gait, and narrow is the way, that leadeth unto life, and few there be that find it."

Matthew 7

New Ways to Cope with Stress

By Robert Marin

Hippocrates said to look to the spine for the solution ...
I was walking along the halls of a recent health and lifestyle expo where you can see all the latest fads on weight-loss, exercise gear, gym equipment, and super-antioxidants, when I overheard one of the staff ask a passerby: "Would you like to get a stress check up?"

The customer answered, "No thanks, she is standing right next to me", pointing to his wife, then laughed and walked on. Some people think stress is a joke. Other people use it to explain everything that is wrong in their lives and will talk endlessly about how many pills they are on and why they cannot cope.

The problem with stress is that you can't live with it and you cannot escape from it. Stress takes a hold when we are young and it never lets go. The disease becomes entrenched. I use the word dis-ease rather than disease as dis-ease encompasses the whole body, while disease points to a particular condition in the body, ignoring the rest of it.[A] How you handle stress is important – it can stop you in your tracks.

What is stress?

Stress is the way the human body breaks down and repairs[1] (scientists call this homeostasis), and how the body is forced to change by your effort to cope with life. More stress equals less balance. Less balance equals more sickness. More sickness creates even more breakdown.

Louis Pasteur, the scientist who was asked to work out why milk would go off after a short period of time, discovered that bacteria were responsible for causing sickness. But Pasteur said on his death bed that it was not the bacteria but the environment that was all important in regard to whether a person became sick.[2] He was saying that our body is the environment and if we change our body then everything else changes.

Why do we focus on the world around us rather than changing ourselves?

The answer is that it's easier, just ineffective.

The outside world and how we live in it is the trigger that throws our body out of balance. I use the "outside world" and "lifestyle" as interchangeable words to refer to anything that we deal with that is not our own body and mind. Lifestyle is everything and everyone else.

Work can be a battle and every communication involves a stress. Let us look at stress and work. Work encompasses about three quarters of our life.[3] It is an area that is often fraught with daily tensions, straining our emotional life, stirring up fears of scarcity, abandonment, rejection, fear itself and inadequacy.

Despite all the different jobs in the world with their different stresses, the effects in us are similar.

If there are twenty accountants in a room, there would be twenty different opinions about how to cope with the challenges of being an accountant; however the job itself creates similar effects in their bodies. Accountants who are placed under heavy workloads have a tendency towards raised cholesterol. Similarly, you could be an easy-going air traffic controller or an anxious one; nevertheless, air traffic controllers seem to suffer from adrenal fatigue, hypertension, peptic ulcers and cardio vascular problems, because their work is exacting and can involve life threatening situations. Meanwhile, working long hours, irrespective of the different occupational groups, leads to heart incidents.[4] We now know that stress affects you if you think it does, and stress will affect you even if you think it doesn't.

How do we know we are adversely affected by stress?

In the early stages we may not know we have stress as the body is absorbing the pressure, but eventually our body will explode.

The aches and pains you suffer from depend very much on your lifestyle.

Dr Hans Selye, author of the book *The Stress of Life*, wrote there is a special way that stress causes the body to deteriorate, involving your musculoskeletal system then into your digestive system then weakening of the immune system and then attacking the cardio vascular system.[5]

The body tells us when stress has become excessive. Resistance to change is a big factor for many people and we have learned that this sort of stress affects the brain and can cause depression, digestive problems, sleep disorders, back pain, circulation problems and high blood pressure.

If you are the type of person who listens to the warning signs you may notice snoring, getting hot at night in bed, hot feet, perspiration after eating a meal, waking up tired and or in pain, poor sex drive and/or sleep patterns, lack of desire to exercise, poor memory.

All or any of these symptoms are simply your body's alert system, letting you know that you are under stress.[6]

The good news is that changing the way you "do your life" can influence how stress affects you. Cancer used to be considered a genetic problem, but now the majority of cancers are considered to be due to lifestyle and therefore influenced by stress.[7] *We become aware that how we live is in our control.*

Here is what happened to me.

I recall about twenty five years ago I had the opportunity of seeing my parents' spines on x-rays when they were about fifty years of age. I remember seeing degenerative changes on the bones and discs, what most would call arthritis; they both had poorly formed spinal curvatures with my mother having a scoliosis (a sideways curvature when it should be straight, while looking at the spine from the front). My father had high blood pressure and gout. Neither suffered chronic back pain although both had visited chiropractors for acute episodes of back pain. My mother was gluten and lactose intolerant.

Not long after graduating from RMIT University in Victoria ,Australia. I suffered from chronic fatigue. I had major digestive problems and my immune system was dealing with one cold after another and I could not get enough sleep. It seemed I had inherited all the negative traits of both parents.

Twenty five years later, my spine is now a normal shape (no longer possessing any family spinal traits) with no evidence of arthritis and no bone or disc deformity. My fatigue is gone and my immunity is back to normal, and this has occurred at the age my parents were when I first saw 'those' x-rays.

What separates us from the animal kingdom is our ability to educate ourselves and our ability to change what and how we think. Understanding how the world around us works and feeling safe in it is a primary need for survival.[8] Changing your deepest held beliefs about the world, changes your life accordingly. Your health is based on your beliefs.

One's destination is never a place, rather a way of looking at things.

HENRY MILLER

The statement above doesn't mean you can think what you like and it will come true. You cannot just think something is not stressful and it becomes so. Understanding that we are more in control of what happens in our body and therefore able to create better health by our actions can give us a better life.

What do we need to change in our thinking?

Let us look at our life and health in a new way. Diseases like heart disease, arthritis, hyperinsulinemia and hypoglycemia (precursors to diabetes), and cancers that are particularly associated with aging in our society, have so far eluded a solution.[9]

The new model of health and medicine

1. The whole is greater than the sum of its parts.
   (Old model: the whole is equal to its parts)

2. Each part is representative of the whole (like a hologram).
   (Old model: parts can be removed without affecting the whole)

3. Matter is a complex aggregate of molecules within a specialised energy field.
   (Old model: there is only matter, no energy field)

4. Interference within the energy field can alter the function of the matter.

5. Our energy field is affected by our thoughts, emotions, diet, pollution, physical trauma, and electromagnetic disturbances – and this interference alters our matter, our body.

Simply stated, *anything and everything affects everything and anything.*

So, in order to make the best use of the new model and improve our health, we need to be able to measure stress in our body, irrespective of where it started. If this measurement was mathematical, like measuring the force loads needed to keep a bridge from collapsing, then it would be easy for us to see. If we could see it, we might understand it. In order to measure these stresses, we need something or someone to compare normal with abnormal.[10] Surprisingly, finding an optimally well person has been a difficult process. It was not until scientists at NASA studied the optimal shape for the spine in designing the best position to withstand the forces of space travel that the normal spine shape was confirmed. Their spine has an "S" shape from the side, and "straight vertical shape" when looking front on – just as we see in the text books, which is convenient. We can leave the minute details for another time.[11]

Not all stresses are the same.

There is one stress which affects us all, irrespective of our job or lifestyle. It is Gravity Stress. With gravity stress you cannot predict that you are going to get heart problems or ulcers but it never leaves you alone, not even for a second. Gravity stress can take years to develop its effect while our whole being is consumed with resisting it. It is doubly worse if you spend the day sitting in an office chair.[12] Do you remember seeing people as they age getting shorter, getting stooped, walking with a shuffle. Do you see people tripping over small irregularities on the footpath? Gravity stress is responsible.

Chiropractors call the early stages of this "forward head posture". This is where your head is sitting forward of your shoulders. The problem starts when we are very young, copying our parents and their posture, learning to walk as babies, carrying heavy bags to school, sitting at school and in front of computers.

Nevertheless, it is a stress like any other and therefore it has a solution.

As well as standing correctly against the force of gravity stress, there is moving correctly. Movement is how we survive. It is normal to move well.

What's the problem with how we move? Moving is not just putting one foot in front of the other. You are unlikely to recognise if you are not moving well as there is no immediate sign. Our brain makes us move – moving is supposed to be automatic, without any conscious effort on our part. The key to a healthy life is found in how we move. The problem is you cannot move well if the spine is not aligned and shaped well.[13]

Two of my chiropractic mentors who were pioneers in this field of stress analysis were Dr Donald Harrison and Dr Lowell Ward.

Dr Harrison discovered that the further from a "normal" shape we find the position of the spine, the greater the effect stress is having on us and the less we are coping.

With the new model of health, stress can be measured and its effects reduced by correcting the structure of the spine, just as you would alter the shape of a bridge or building to better withstand the effects of gravity. Therefore, by returning the spine to its normal shape, stress can be reduced in the body.[14] This also reduces the tension the brain has to process, which thereby positively affects the rest of the body. Reducing the stress we have in our body and through the nervous system alters the stress our brain receives.

Dr Ward then took Dr Harrison's principle of spine measurements and found out how our lifestyles, emotions, and mental stresses affected our health and created the technique called MESA (Mental Emotional Structural Analysis) to analyse the stress in our spine, correct the dis-ease in our body and restore balance.[14]

What results have we achieved with this new way of seeing?

These doctors who study stress, both medical and chiropractic, therefore see the spine and the effect it has on our body differently from therapists who are simply searching for ways to relieve pain. The example below was some of Dr Ward's analysis in action.

Jake was less than two years old when I first met him and had been diagnosed autistic by medical doctors. We adjusted him for six weeks with little change. We tested Jakes mother who had a similar spinal pattern but no autistic issues, and started her under care. Six weeks later, Jake is responding to care. Jake has been normal ever since. How does adjusting Jake and his mother together create this change in condition. Incidentally, Jake's aunt and grandmother all had similar spinal patterns. Can stress patterns be passed on through families? The short answer to this is yes. I do not mean only through genetics but also through lifestyle. People who spend enough time with each other, eat the same foods and sit in the same chairs, will develop similar problems. Children model themselves on their parents, see the world similarly and therefore develop similar patterns. If you are old enough you may remember the song 'Cats in the Cradle' where the father recognises that his son grew up to be just like him, never having the time to just stop and spend some time.

A plan to help reduce stress and the negative effects in your body

1. Have your spine measured for stress and then have its shape restored to normal. Chiropractic helps restore the balance and, in turn, removes the obstacle for the body to repair itself.

2. After your spine is back to its normal shape see your chiropractor regularly to make sure you keep it that way.

3. Decide what you want for your health in twenty years and find a chiropractor you can work with who can help you create that.

4. Don't be casual in dealing with problems now; second chances are rare.

5. Look at your issues and only take on what you need to.

6. Understand how your body works. Ensure your chiropractor includes education as part of your correction plan; this reduces the resistance that may occur when internal changes happen. Knowledge creates safety.

Chiropractors also say, *"Look to the spine."*

CHAPTER 32

*"What lies behind us and what lies before us
are tiny matters compared to what lies within us"*

Ralph Waldo Emerson

Headaches are a Sign

By Wayne Whittingham

Headaches (HA), are they just a part of modern life? So many people seem to think so. As a doctor of chiropractic, so many times during an initial consultation I have had this exchange with patients:

"Do you suffer with HAs?" (Doctor)

"Oh yeah, just the usual; usually because I am tired, or too many hours on the computer, it's my husband, the boss, the kids ..." (Patient)

No, it's an alarm bell; the dashboard light on your car warning you that there is something wrong. We don't ignore a warning light on a car (which is disposable), yet we treat our bodies differently – we take a painkiller. Will pulling over and unscrewing your dashboard light or putting a band aid over it make it go away? Of course not! That may sound ridiculous, but that's what we do with our bodies instead of getting to the bottom of the problem. It's a lovely journey, getting to understand your body, how it works and why things can play up. This chapter is about explaining this concept in clearly understandable terms; how and why HAs can plague your life or, worse still, take over your life. I have spent the past 18 years trying to better understand and manage patients HAs, so for those who suffer from chronic HAs, this chapter is for you.

Ivan Illich once said that culture makes pain tolerable by interpreting its necessity; only pain perceived as curable is intolerable. In my experience, I would say that is also true of most HAs. The majority of HAs are benign, meaning that they have no sinister underlying cause, and people regularly suffering HAs often make an excuse for them or attribute them to something in their day, ranging from fatigue to stress or hunger; the list is endless. The problem with this line of thinking is that the sufferer will take medication and continue suffering from HAs without ever thinking that there might be an underlying cause; and, let's face it, HAs are so common.

In fact, they are one of the most common reasons people go to doctors, one of the most common conditions that people seek medication for and one of the most common reasons leading to drug dependency and analgesic abuse.

Some relevant headache facts:

- Headaches are the most prevalent ailment of mankind.

- Up to 75% of males and 80% of females are affected by HAs in any one year period.

- On average, a HA sufferer has his or her condition for 15 years before entering treatment in specialist HA clinics, when cost of medication and treatment are combined they are enormous. These patients spend between $500 and $1000 a year on their HA problem, after the cost of the initial diagnostic evaluation.

HAs which have their origin in the cervical spine (neck) are now reported by some specialists to be one of the most common forms of chronic benign HAs; in simple terms, the neck is one of the most common causes of HAs. (10% of people who see a chiropractor, do so for HAs.)

When diagnostic tests have been exhausted and the brain scans, MRI and allergy testing all come up negative, the HA sufferer is left searching for relief. This chapter is focused on providing fascinating insights into new sources and cures for the seemingly incurable HA.

Understanding what causes headaches and where they may originate from, will lead to a better understanding about how chiropractic can help.

HEADACHE TYPES

Structural

Although now reported to be one of the most common HA types, this is still the most overlooked and, unfortunately for the HA sufferer, often missed. HA sufferers commonly think to have their eyes checked, even dental and temporomandibular joint problems (jaw) are addressed, but until recently, faults in the spine and skull were overlooked.

According to the British Association for the Study of Headaches (2007) guidelines, 15% of the UK population have migraines, and a staggering 80% have episodic tension-type headaches. There is a 98% higher prevalence in women than in men, and headaches are the most common reason for attending a general practice surgery or a neurology clinic.

Cranial complex

The adult skull consists of 28 bones. The larger bones (cranial bones) are joined together by sutures. In the past, many anatomists and doctors thought that these sutures were immovable joints.

Movement of the teeth and the accompanying cranial bone changes may place stresses within the skeletal structure without any obvious immediate symptoms. These structural imbalances will cause the body to be in a constant, active adaptive state; this, in turn, can put stress on the central nervous system.

Cranial bone motion was discovered in 1939 by William Sutherland (an osteopath). During cranial motion, the 28 cranial bones function as a unit; the rhythmic micro-motion occurs within a physiological range of six to twelve cycles per minute, i.e. the brain, along with the sacrum in the pelvis, pumps cerebral spinal fluid around the spinal cord and brain. The cranial dura compartmentalises the brain and furnishes it with a duct system (venous and cerebral spinal fluid) for irrigation, nourishment and waste removal. Both cranial bone and dural membrane motion provide a synchronous pumping action that supports cerebral spinal fluid flow and ensures the health of the central nervous system (CNS).

The dural membrane passes through the base of the skull, attaches to the first three cervical vertebrae (top three bones in the neck) and continues down the spinal cord and attaches to the sacrum. Unfortunately, people whose body structures have been traumatised through the birth process (forceps delivery, prolonged labour), physical trauma, whiplash injuries, fractures, difficult dental extractions or surgical operations, will have a great likelihood of structural torqueing or twisting of muscles, ligaments and other body structures. This, in turn, can create torque in the spinal dura, which is transmitted up into the skull. This causes the cranial bones and sutures to become jammed, ultimately resulting in HAs.

If one visualises the dural tube, which connects the pelvis and skull, as a towel that becomes twisted and shortened, then one can understand how the cranial dura will pull to one side. All cranial nerves pass through the cranial dura. If the dura is under tension (or torque), then the nerves passing through will be affected and neurological symptoms will appear, HAs being one of the earliest signs. Because cranial principles are not taught at university level, most orthodontists, neurologists and other health care professionals do not possess the knowledge needed to recognise the source of the problem and properly treat the patient.

Scientists have documented the existence of nerves, blood vessels and connecting fibres in the structural areas and anatomists have also shown the direct physical connection between the inside and outside of the skull. The dural membrane that surrounds the brain communicates with and influences the outside of the skull by means of an outer fibrous layer. This layer passes through the sutures and covers bony portions of the skull. For this reason, internal tensions have the potential to cause external changes such as muscle spasms and vice-type pressure. The reverse is also true; whether the HA is due to physical tension or a vascular migraine, the dural membranes will be affected.

As these dural membranes are innervated by cervical and cranial nerves they too can become the source of HA pain.

Robinson (1995) identified a previously undocumented anatomical connection between the "rectus capitus posterior minor" muscle (small back muscle) and the "dura mater" (the tough fibrous membrane covering the brain and the spinal cord and lining the inner surface of the skull). A band of fibrous connective tissue extends from this muscle to the spinal dura between the atlas (top bone in the neck) and the occiput (bottom of the skull). If traction is applied to the muscle, traction on the spinal dura transmitting to the cranial dura will result, and may cause headaches (as the dura mater is a pain-sensitive structure).

The source of migraine HA is generally vascular, whereby the larger arteries and veins in the skull dilate while the smaller vessels that carry the blood from the arteries to the veins constrict. The overall affect is engorgement of the larger arteries and veins, resulting in a build-up of blood within the skull. The blood is restricted from leaving the skull by spasm of the muscles at the base of the skull. This reciprocal action is the body's attempt to counteract the problem. However, the greater the dilation the greater the reciprocal constriction of the smaller blood vessels, and even though there is an excess of blood in the brain, the quantity reaching parts of the brain is diminished. This is what causes the pounding head and other various neurological symptoms associated with migraine HAs. The other symptoms usually associated with migraines arise because three cranial nerves exit at the base of the skull. These nerves have extensive innervations to many vital body areas.

The glosso-pharyngeal (ninth cranial nerve) accounts for the changes in taste and swallowing. The vagus nerve (tenth) can affect the voice box, heart, lungs, stomach, liver, spleen, kidneys, pancreas and intestines. The eleventh cranial nerve affects the neck muscles which go into spasm, which further perpetuates the problem.

I'm going to get technical here but it is important to understand the mechanism in order to find a solution.

As the structural distortions progress, the dural pressures will begin to restrict the flow of cerebral spinal fluid (CSF) into the brain tissue. The early visual symptoms result from the visual centres of the brain being deprived of their normal quantities of blood and CSF. As toxic metabolic waste accumulates neurological dysfunctions start to arise. Increased intercranial distortions will cause excessive stimulation of the parasympathetic portion of the nervous system; this in turn causes an increase in production of CSF from the ventricles of the brain. This causes a further increase in intercranial pressure, alongside the increase in pressure from the reduction of blood flow exiting the brain. The chain of events that set off the dural torqueing will cause the atlas vertebrae to distort; this is commonly referred to by chiropractors as a "subluxation of the atlas". The dural torqueing can result from a single or various combinations of structural distortions such as the pelvis, spinal vertebrae, dental malocclusion or cranial bone restrictions. These structural problems can be triggered by emotional, physical, nutritional or physiological stressors.

Cervicogenic

Until recently, these were probably the most overlooked of the headaches and, as a consequence, the most commonly mistreated – the primary reason being that, as mentioned earlier, until research conducted in the 1960s, doctors and scientists did not believe that the cranial bones moved. Similarly, until the 1980s most doctors and scientists did not believe the neck could be the source of HAs. The work of Nikolai Bogduk (an anatomist) showed the mechanism by which the neck causes pain referred into the head.

Nerves that exit from the upper part of the neck send messages into the brainstem. The brainstem also receives messages from the Trigeminal nerve (cranial nerve five), which supplies the face. Because the area in the brainstem (trigeminocervical nucleus) is more familiar with receiving messages from the trigeminal nerve, when it receives messages from the neck structures, it cannot decipher if these messages are from the head or neck region; hence, due to familiarity, it perceives the source of the pain to be in the facial region.

The reason these headaches are so common is due to our modern day lifestyles. Many of us are much less active than our previous generation: we rely on our cars more, more people sit at work all day and children and adults spend a lot of time in front of computers for work and play, and there is the added stress and pressure of our ever-expanding consumer world. All these factors put stress on the spine. For some, this may even have started at childbirth.

Dr Fryman, an osteopath, conducted a study on 1250 new born infants. He reported that 10% of the newborns had severe visual trauma inflicted on their heads; this may have occurred in utero or during labour. Cranial examination on the remaining infants revealed cranial bone strains in 78% of the cases. The study concluded that nearly 90% of all infants had cranial distortions that occurred while they were being carried or during delivery.

If allowed to go untreated, these distortions have the potential of causing structural imbalances that can be the source of chronic HAs and other neurological problems that occur during adolescence or adulthood.

Like snowflakes, no two headaches are the same, and the longer one suffers with headaches the greater the likelihood that secondary headaches can arise. Most benign headache sufferers lie somewhere along the 'headache continuum model': this model was proposed by Waters (1973) and unites the two broad categories of migraine and tension headache into a category forming a continuum. This theory expresses a common underlying pathology as opposed to two distinct pathophysiological entities.

NUTRITIONAL ASPECTS OF HEADACHES

Nutrition is an enormous topic, and the essentials of proper nutrition are covered in more detail in other areas of this book, but taking note of how food affects your body could be vital in preventing future headaches.

The brain differs from all the other organs in the body in that it is solely nourished by sugar (glucose), and consequently is the most sensitive to change in sugar levels. Studies have shown that the level of blood sugar controls the amount of electrical activity in the brain. The ingestion of refined sugars will cause a jump in sugar levels in the blood stream and consequently cause a rapid increase in insulin. This scenario of sugar highs and lows puts a huge stress on the brain. In its simplest form, a junk food diet, which is lacking in many essential nutrients, will have a major impact on normal brain function, commonly resulting in HAs.

In relation to the digestive system and HAs, one is better off to have a diet high in complex carbohydrates. By having a diet high in roughage, one maintains healthier muscular tone of the intestinal wall and more efficiency expelling toxic wastes. By preventing toxic waste build up, one preserves the normal bacterial flora, which produces B complex vitamins, vitamin K and glutamic acid (essential for brain function), and regulates the normal flora to convert carbohydrates to lactic acid. The lactic acid promotes growth of other healthy bacteria and restricts the growth of toxin-producing organisms. Lactic acid is responsible for the regulation of guanidine, which is one of the most toxic products in the body, and a cause of toxic HAs.

A healthy digestive system will also prevent the release of histamine in the bowel, which is a dilator of blood vessels, and can cause histamine HA.

Some of the most common substances thought to cause HAs are:

1. **Caffeine** – Has a direct effect on the blood vessels. Very commonly, heavy caffeine consumers find their dependency increases and there comes a point when without the caffeine they develop HAs.

2. **Sodium nitrate or nitrite** – Very commonly used in packaged or processed meats, it is also found in spinach, beets, radishes and lettuce. It's also said to have a direct effect on blood vessels.

3. **MSG (mono sodium glutamate)** – Used as a flavour enhancer, it is commonly used in restaurants and take-away food. MSG causes HAs to come on quite quickly after eating. People who are sensitive to MSG are usually susceptible to migraines and other vascular HAs.

4. **Alcohol and histamine** – When combined, they have a strong vaso-dilating effect on the blood vessels. Alcohol provokes HAs within 30–45 minutes, the time it takes to dilate arterioles. Alcohol also causes histamine release from the body, which causes an increased heart rate and, at higher doses, flushing and vascular HAs. Red wine is the most common alcoholic drink to have a high histamine content and is renowned for causing HAs in individuals who suffer migraine or cluster HAs. Other sources rich in histamine include beer, fermented foods (e.g. sauerkraut), and chocolate; these all contain enough histamine to induce HAs. Foods that release histamine include egg whites, strawberries, tomatoes, citrus fruits, shell fish and alcohol.

5. **Vasoactive amines** – foods containing serotonin, tryptamine, dopamine and norepinephrine include avocados, bananas, plums, oranges, pineapples, fermented cheeses, pickled herrings, salt dried fish and wine. Individuals with diet-related migraines have lower levels of a platelet enzyme (phenolsulphotransferase) that breaks down these products. Red wine contains inhibitors of phenolsulphotransferase. Phenylethylamine is also a vasoactive amine and is found in chocolate, cheese and red wines, all renowned for precipitating migraines.

6. **Too much vitamin A** – A chronic high dosage can cause an increase in intercranial pressure; this will cause a HA.

7. **Drugs** – Almost all drugs in the current British National Formulary (BNF), list HA as a possible side-effect. Therefore, any medication that a HA sufferer is taking could be a possible trigger. Chronic HA sufferers who become addicted to painkillers may be causing their own head pain. Heavy consumption on a daily basis will maintain the blood vessels in a constricted state. By withdrawing from the painkillers, dilation of the blood vessels occurs, which can trigger a HA, so failure to meet your daily quota of these substances may trigger a rebound HA.

8. **Birth control pills** – the PILL changes the female hormone balance. As more research is coming to light on the effect of hormones and HAs, it is becoming clear that any artificial alteration of this delicate balance can lead to a host of unpredictable symptoms, including HAs.

9. **Tyramine** – again dilates blood vessels and has a potential to trigger allergic HAs. It is commonly found in red wine and aged cheeses, processed meats and marinated/pickled food.

10. **Salt** – some foods have a high salt content, or salt is used in the preparation, e.g. pork, bacon, salted crisps, nuts and many processed foods. Excessive salt (sodium chloride) increases blood volume, which causes cells to retain fluids. This increases the blood pressure, so the arteries have to dilate to counter this effect, and this can be a cause of HAs.

Citrus fruits can cause HAs in some people who have an enzyme deficiency. The enzymes they lack are necessary for neutralising amines in foods. Some foods have large quantities of amines and, without the enzyme, HAs (and even migraines) can be triggered.

Other foods listed by migraine and HA sufferers include:

- Peanuts and peanut butter
- Pizza
- Potatoes, chips
- Fresh fruits, e.g. kiwi fruit, plums and raspberries
- Bread and crackers

One new theory is that craving certain foods could also signal an oncoming migraine. These kinds of migraines are also made more unpredictable because eating the food may not trigger pain every time, and because often other trigger factors are also required, like bright lights or stress.

A food HA diary is the most valuable way to determine which foods, if any, relate to your HA. At least two weeks of complete avoidance is necessary before the relationship is clear. Remember that many substances or combination of foods can trigger HAs. If you have HAs frequently, you should avoid all of the above foods. If the HAs improve by avoiding these foods, you can reintroduce one at a time to identify the triggers for you.

As with a migraine, preventing a food headache is only possible when you learn to recognise and avoid the trigger. By ensuring you drink two litres of water a day you should avoid any HA caused by dehydration. Your blood sugars are the other factor that can cause HAs, common when you haven't eaten enough.

Certain HAs do require immediate medical attention; these include: severe, sudden HAs that seems to come on like a "bolt of lightning", HAs accompanied by a loss of consciousness, alterations of sensations, confusion, visual blurring or other neurological changes (e.g. change in the pupils), HAs which come on rapidly and have associated neck stiffness and fever, and HAs which have suddenly changed in character.

Treatment

The clinical picture of HAs that usually respond best to manual therapy are – primarily a unilateral HA which seems to be getting worse with time; pain is usually located around the eye or at the base of the skull, with concomitant neck pain; the HA pain can often be severe and described as stabbing or pulsating, and can lead to vomiting; dizziness, nausea and shoulder stiffness are also common; and in between HA episodes, neck pain with associated tension and stiffness (usually the person is aware that the HA is coming on, which may be initiated by head and neck movements, pressure applied to the base of the skull, holding the head in a sustained posture, or stress).

Idealistic management for chronic benign disabling HAs may achieve better long-term results by combining both medical and chiropractic skills and perspective. The earlier the detection of abnormal spinal mechanics (especially following head or neck trauma), the better the treatment outcome will be.

From a biomechanical perspective, it would appear logical that any HA that has persisted for many years, in some instances decades, will develop a cascade of pathophysiological functions. Neuroanatomical connections that exit within the vicinity of the brain stem can potentially cause tension in the cervical musculature. Hence it only seems reasonable that massage may provide temporary relief, by interrupting the above cascade of pathophysiological functions. The degree of pain relief will inevitably depend upon the extent to which the muscular components contribute to the overall HA picture.

Alarming facts (Granella1987):

- Traditional medical management of HAs placed heavy reliance on medication. This has had significant harmful effects.

- The most frequent reason for the abuse of analgesics appears to be headache.

- The largest single factor favouring the transformation of episodic HA into a chronic HA is drug abuse.

Drug therapies have been investigated for chronic headaches (CHAs) with theoretically different approach points; for example: the effects of anti-inflammatory drugs on the prostaglandin system (Sjaastad 1990), oxygen on the vascular system, sumatriptan on ergotamine (Bovim 1993, Martelleti 1993), and morphine on the CNS pain perception (Bovim 1993). These studies have revealed that these medications have little or no effect on the HA symptoms, with the exception of morphine, which provided temporary relief. However, this is not an ethical long-term solution as it is simply a powerful analgesic.

The surgical approaches investigated include transecting the C2 nerve route (Jansen 1989), or major and minor occipital nerves (Jansen and Markakis 1989). Also, radio frequency treatment of the periosteum of the occipital bone has been attempted (Blume 1985); however these have not had positive effects in most patients. These surgical approaches also suffer from a high percentage of HA reoccurrence. Unfortunately, these results are usually based on case studies and are not tested under trial conditions. Due to the poor outcome and invasive nature of these treatments they should be considered as a last resort in cases which have not responded to other non invasive therapeutic approaches.

> *As a HA sufferer, you have to be aware that if a structural problem exists, no amount of drugs or surgical intervention will resolve the HA.*

When a structural problem exists, correction should best be performed by spinal and/or cranial adjustment techniques that focus on correcting the biomechanics.

Chiropractors have defined structural faults as vertebral subluxations complex (VSC) or biomechanical joint dysfunction. The essential elements of these entities include:

- Abnormal function (movement) in a spinal joint (motion segment)
- Neurological and vascular involvement (vasomotor)
- Frequently, but not necessarily, a structural (static) displacement of the vertebrae.

It is essentially a functional entity, involving restricted vertebral movement in one or more planes of motion. However, unless there is a structural misalignment, VSC cannot be seen on x-ray.

There is a growing body of evidence in the medical literature to indicate that chiropractors and osteopaths are the best equipped to perform the highly skilled spinal and/or cranial adjustments that are required to address these mechanical faults.

Chiropractors use a wholistic approach. The treatment program prescribed by chiropractors involves:

- Restoration of normal spinal function to a previously immobilised joint using a diverse range of manual adjustive techniques to relieve the altered neurophysiology
- Postural advice
- Dietary advice – avoidance of certain foods
- Exercise recommendations
- Soft tissue therapy to surrounding musculature
- Referral for further assessment or other specialist services – such as

biofeedback, counselling and/or medication (which may be given in conjunction with the chiropractic treatment) – for psychological factors identified in the history.

Headaches are NOT a normal part of modern day living, they are a symptom that something is wrong. Sadly, we often ignore them and medicate the pain. If you suffer from chronic headaches it makes sense to rule out that your spine is not the cause. For this you need to consult a registered chiropractor.

CHAPTER 33

"There are two ways to live your life – one is as though nothing is a miracle, the other is as though everything is a miracle."

Albert Einstein

Arthritis – Help is at Hand

By Rob Sandford

Over 9 million people in the UK suffer with arthritis[1] and in Australia 3.85 million, whilst more than 21% of Americans (46.4 million) have arthritis or a similar rheumatic (joint related) condition.[2,3] By 2030 the number of sufferers is expected to rise to 67 million in the United States (US) – a 41% increase – and it is already the main cause of disability in the US.[2,3] Surprisingly, the statistics also indicate that nearly two thirds of arthritis sufferers are under 65 years old.[2,3]

Clearly, arthritis represents one of the most significant threats to health, mobility and quality of life in the western world and finding an effective solution or management strategy is vital. Better still, of course, would be an understanding of how to prevent arthritis.

Arthritis is actually a group of conditions involving damage to the joints of the body, causing pain, swelling and stiffness. There are, in fact, more than 100 different types of arthritis which can be further divided into three main types: Osteoarthritis – often considered to be age or trauma related; Inflammatory Arthritis – most commonly the result of auto-immune disease; and Septic Arthritis – caused by infection within the joint.

Even these categories are groups of diseases though, and the clinical picture of each individual case can be quite varied.

Osteoarthritis (OA) and Rheumatoid Arthritis (RA) – a common form of Inflammatory Arthritis – are the most widespread types.

Osteoarthritis

Osteoarthritis is the most common form of arthritis, affecting approximately 8 million people in the UK.[4]

OA, also described as degenerative joint disease (DJD), involves the breakdown of the joint – particularly the cartilage lining the bones. As the body struggles against the damage, immune system reaction and regrowth processes can further accelerate the damage.[5] When the surfaces of the bone become less well protected by cartilage, the bone itself can become exposed and damaged. The regrowth of bone in response leads to thick areas of bone in the central area of the bone surfaces (*eburnation*) and bone spur formation at the edges of the joint (*osteophytes*).

The sufferer experiences increasing pain, swelling and stiffness, especially with weight bearing (including walking and standing). As a result of decreased movement because of the pain, regional muscles may also waste, and ligaments may become looser.[6]

OA is commonly referred to as "wear and tear" of the joints and therefore often considered to be both the result of age and a normal response to ageing. This description is unhelpful though as neither is strictly true.

In our society we have developed a habit of replacing the word "common" with the word "normal". In other words, when something happens a lot it gets referred to as normal. For example, it is very common for women to suffer period pain, but does that make it normal? It is common for people to suffer hayfever symptoms in the springtime, but is this normal? It is also common for us to develop high blood pressure as we age, but does this mean it is normal? If any of these things were normal, it would mean that people who did not suffer period pain, hayfever or high blood pressure would be abnormal or unhealthy! Therefore, although arthritis is common, it isn't normal.

It also isn't accurate to blame OA on age. In contrast to Rheumatoid arthritis, the degenerative changes associated with OA are characterised as being asymmetrical. That is to say, in most cases, symptoms are present in a joint on one side of the body, but not (or not as severely) in the same joint on the other side of the body. Chiropractors often note that the OA in a client's right knee for example cannot be the result of age, since both the knees are the same age and the left knee does not show the same changes! Obviously there must be more at work than just "so-called normal" age-related wear and tear.

Statistics do show that the incidence of arthritis increases with age and you become more likely to suffer arthritic changes later in life. It is estimated that 80% of the US population will have x-ray evidence of OA by age 65, although only 60% will have symptoms.[7] However, all chiropractors have seen x-rays of clients of advanced age with little or no degenerative or arthritic changes.

The increased likelihood of OA as you grow older results from the build up of minor damage and dysfunction to the joint over the years. It is a process that takes time to develop. Since most of us collect minor joint damage and dysfunction through our lives it becomes very common to get arthritis as we age – but it isn't normal. The more damage and dysfunction there is, the earlier the arthritis occurs. So what is the damage and dysfunction and how does it happen?

In very real terms, the health of the joints in your body relies on their movement. After all, the joints were designed for the purpose of movement. If this stops it is easy to see that the joint would immediately become less healthy.

Picture the pond in your back garden. In order to maintain the clear water and health of the pond, most garden ponds use a pump. This makes sure that the water is kept flowing and the steady exchange of important nutrients and waste products occur. This is particularly vital for the fish living in your pond that depend on the flushing in of the nutrients and food and flushing out of the waste products.

If you were to turn the pump off for a significant period of time the lack of water movement and resultant cycle of exchange would cause a build-up of bacteria and algae and a very unhealthy environment for your fish. The stagnant pond is a terrific analogy for what occurs within your joints if movement is lacking or if the appropriate or full movement is no longer possible.

In simple terms, each of the moving joints of your body comprises two bone ends covered in cartilage. Between the two bone ends is a gap filled with fluid. The whole joint is then surrounded by a sac called a synovial membrane. The synovial fluid (the fluid within the sac) acts just like the pond, feeding and nourishing the joint surfaces and collecting the waste. Movement of the joint performs the same job as the pump in your pond, creating movement of the fluid and an exchange of the joint nutrients and joint waste. A lack of movement within the joint literally allows the synovial fluid to become stagnant and less healthy. The result is reduced health of the joint surfaces and structures.[8]

A lack of movement is one of the major results of changes in the alignment of the bones which form the joint. In chiropractic, a misalignment of the joints of the spine is referred to as a "vertebral subluxation". This is particularly important because of the vital role the spine plays in protecting the spinal cord and spinal nerves. It is thought that changes in the alignment can create nerve interference and the performance of the body is reduced as a consequence. However, the joint movement is also reduced and if this continues over a long period of time stagnation occurs and the joint itself starts to degenerate. Thus, not only is your performance impaired, but the likelihood of OA increases.

Any joint within the body can become misaligned, when it is referred to simply as a joint subluxation. Chiropractors are trained to locate and correct these subluxations, to restore proper nerve function and normal movement. Chiropractors tend to focus on the vertebral subluxation because of the importance of the spinal cord, but are able to correct subluxations throughout the body. By restoring the proper motion in the joint, effectively, "the pump" is turned on and over time the health of the joint can increase.

Distortion, disruption or damage to the joint caused by significant traumas or subtle misalignment can also lead to arthritis in the area.

The joint can be compared to a complex piece of engineering, specifically and precisely designed for its purpose – movement.

Any change to the structures within the joint, the distribution of weight, or forces through the joint, affects this precise design. The resulting alteration in the mechanics or motion of the joint can be important.

As a comparison, you can imagine that if you were to hop on one foot for 4 hours a day for 6 months, one shoe would wear out quicker than the other! Distortion or changes to the joint surface create the same abnormal wear, leading to osteoarthritis.

Major traumas, such as ski falls, motorbike crashes or sports injuries, can obviously cause this joint distortion and lead to osteoarthritis later in life.

However, minor traumas (particularly repetitive traumas) and minor changes to the joint can also play a part in OA. These may be the result of postural alterations or changes in alignment caused by joint subluxation.

For example, subluxation of the lower back joints will cause disruption and reduced movement in the spinal joints, but also cause the distribution of weight through the hips and legs to change. It is likely that one hip will be supporting slightly more weight than the other. It is suspected that over time this will lead to increased degeneration on one side.

Chiropractic is a very effective pain management tool, but in addition, by correcting the vertebral subluxation, chiropractors not only restore the normal movement within the joint but also the proper joint forces, alignment and weight distribution. This can radically impact the progression of arthritis and even prevent the degeneration occurring.

Rheumatoid Arthritis

Rheumatoid arthritis (RA) is the most common form of auto-immune arthritis. In auto-immune diseases like this, for an unknown reason the body starts to attack itself. With RA the attack is not limited to the joints but involves other tissue cells as well. However, the most damage often occurs in the linings of the joint and the cartilage surfaces of the bone within the joint. It can eventually spread to involve the bone surfaces themselves.

The synovial membrane encasing the joint becomes inflamed and the amount of fluid within the joint increases. As the process progresses, the cartilage covering the bone surfaces is destroyed and eventually the joint can become fused and immobile. Just as in OA, the main symptoms are pain, swelling and stiffness but also deformity in later stages. The joints affected by RA are often symmetrical and it is also characterised by periods of relative calmness followed by more acute periods of symptoms or inflammatory flare-ups.

The exact cause of RA is unknown and although there appears to be hereditary factors involved, it is largely regarded as an auto-immune process.

The function of the immune system is to protect the body. The immune system works hard to identify threats, both internally and externally, and deal with them. External threats include bacteria and viruses, and examples of internal threats are when the body makes an abnormal or damaged cell. In both cases the role of the immune system is to identify the threat and destroy it.

In the case of an auto-immune disease, rather than destroying threatening cells the body starts to attack healthy cells. As such it is a breakdown of the detection process. The body begins to see non-threatening cells as threats. This can have devastating effects as the immune system is very powerful and effective. It is also difficult to stop as the immune system will continue until the (perceived) threat is gone.

At the moment, the only way to treat these conditions is to use drugs to suppress or quieten the immune system. The weakness of this is that the effect of these drugs is indiscriminate. In other words, they affect all of the immune system, not a small part. Therefore, with a reduced immune system the body becomes less able to protect itself against real threats.

The immune system, like every part of the body, is controlled and regulated by the nerve system. It is conceivable that the breakdown in the threat detection system in particular may occur as a result of reduced nerve function to the important immune system cells; therefore it may be possible that vertebral subluxation and the resultant nerve impairment plays a role in this dysfunction.

Scientific evidence is limited but there are numerous individual case studies which demonstrate significant symptomatic improvement with chiropractic care.[9] Most chiropractors have success stories to tell.

Managing arthritis

Largely, the structural changes to the joint caused by arthritis are considered permanent. However, a body of research suggests that it is possible to stop much of the degeneration caused by OA and even reverse it with chiropractic care.[10–13]

Chiropractic care is certainly proving to be not only effective but increasingly popular. An investigation in 1999 revealed that 63% of people who visited a rheumatologist for osteoarthritis, rheumatoid arthritis or a similar condition, also visited some form of alternative health therapist. Of the alternative therapists consulted, the most common was a chiropractor (31%). More significant, however, was the fact that 73% of those that utilised chiropractic found it helpful.[14]

Unfortunately, once the joint surfaces and structures have degenerated to a certain point, they will never fully recover. Although cartilage regeneration is possible, bone spurs will not shrink away and some changes to the joint will be permanent. Therefore, preventing arthritis is far more effective than treating it.

Put simply, preventing arthritis is best achieved by avoiding the factors which contribute to it. By reducing the stresses on the joints, correcting misalignments and maximising the proper movement, the maximum health of the joint is maintained. In combination with a healthy lifestyle, regular chiropractic care to identify and correct subluxations where necessary is the best way I know to do that.

CHAPTER 34

If there is no such thing as space
And all we have is here ...
And no such thing as time
And all we have is now ...
Then between here and now is ... Love
I Love You

Excerpt from *Whispers of Love* by Kathy Rasch

Depressed? Here is the Other Approach

By Kathy Rasch

What an absolute honour it is to have been a chiropractor for the last 19 years! Every day in practice is a day that I witness the amazing inborn potential that lies within us all, and how a chiropractic adjustment can affect every nerve, tissue, organ and cell – allowing the person's true magnificence to shine. Working with a patient's innate intelligence, respecting that intelligence as highest priority with a focus on freeing rather than controlling and assisting rather than intruding, is the chiropractic way. Miracles happen every day in chiropractic, and over my years in practice I have seen many of my patients with depression and anxiety symptoms experience great improvement.

The effect of a chiropractic adjustment is boundless. It is only restricted by the potential of the human body which, in my opinion, is limitless. Because the nervous system controls every function, freeing that system to operate at its true potential allows all parts of the body to improve. This means on all levels: physical, mental, emotional and spiritual. My passion is working on all these levels with my patients. The potential for healing and growth within the human body is only overshadowed by the unlimited potential of the human spirit. We are incredible beings in so many ways, and yet we all have our story, and our lessons to learn.

There has been much research conducted on the relationship between chiropractic and depression and anxiety. Depression is really a whole body condition that affects body, mind, emotions and spirit. It is not something to be ashamed of, nor is it something you can simply wish away. You can't just "snap out of it" or put on a happy face and think it away. Mood disorders affect over 10% of the population in any given year. The definition from the National Institute of Mental Health is: "A depressive disorder is an illness that involves the body, mood and thoughts. It affects the way a person eats and sleeps, the way one feels about oneself, and the way one thinks about things. A depressive disorder is not the same as a passing blue mood. Without treatment, symptoms can last weeks, months or years."

Clinical Depression, however, is very different to the more general and common feeling of being depressed and/or anxious. Although a low mood or state of dejection that does not affect functioning is often referred to as depression, clinical depression is a clinical diagnosis and may be different from the everyday meaning of "being depressed". Many people identify the feeling of being clinically depressed as "feeling sad for no reason", or "having no motivation to do anything". A person suffering from depression may feel tired, sad, irritable, lazy, unmotivated, and apathetic. Clinical depression often leads to constant negative thinking and sometimes substance abuse. Extreme depression can culminate in its sufferers attempting or committing suicide.

In certain cases, patients can alternate between periods of depression and mania, also known as bipolar disorder or manic depression. Depression (and the fluctuation between depression and mania) is thought to be caused by alterations in serotonin levels in the brain.

While medical science has not determined the exact cause of altered serotonin levels that are suspected to produce depression, recent research has pointed towards a likely trauma-induced origin for certain cases of mood disorders. Evidence supports that trauma (in particular mild concussive injury to the head, neck or upper back) increases the risk of the onset of depression. Following the trauma, mood disorders can be triggered immediately or can take months or years to develop.

The causes of depression though, can vary. Some people carry a genetic predisposition for it, while others begin to experience depression as a result of hormonal imbalances. No matter what the cause may be, one aspect is consistent: there is a change within the brain's chemistry and/or function that allows depression to consume an individual. The good news is that depression can improve with chiropractic. Numerous research studies have documented improvement in depression and related symptoms as a result of chiropractic adjustments which reduce pressure on the brain stem and spinal cord caused by vertebral subluxations.

I'm going to get technical here for a bit but it is necessary in order to show you that what I am saying is researched information and not just anecdotal, so please stay with me.

A research study published in the 7 November 2005 issue of the *Journal of Vertebral Subluxation Research*, showed a positive result in the care of individuals with depression. For the purpose of this study, subjects were selected on the basis of being over 18 years of age and having depression noted in their medical history. Fifteen participants completed the study and were used in determining the results.

In the discussion section of the study, it was noted that the concept of chiropractic care's role in mental health was not a new idea. In fact, it was reported that two major chiropractic psychiatric hospitals functioned successfully for nearly thirty years in Davenport, Iowa. (The 1970s saw a renewed interest in chiropractic care and mental health issues. In 1973, Dr Herman S. Schwartz, a chiropractor, published a book titled *Mental Health and Chiropractic: A Multidisciplinary Approach*. In 1949, Dr Schwartz had published a preliminary report of 350 patients afflicted with a "nervous or mental disorder" and reported that the majority of them showed improvement under chiropractic care).

The subjects of this study were given a standardised test known as the Beck Depression Inventory (aka BDI-II) both before and after receiving specific chiropractic care for correction of subluxations. To be consistent, the same process of analysis and techniques of correction were used in correcting the subluxations determined to be present.

The results showed a significant improvement in the average BDI-II scores of the group. Lower BDI-IIs are considered better than higher scores - the higher the level the more severe the depression. The group as a whole scored a 17 in the BDI-II before chiropractic. After chiropractic care for correction of their subluxations, the group's average score improved to 8. Wow, what amazing results!

The researchers concluded by stating, "This study's results provide support for the hypothesis that a positive relationship exists between a correction of the occipitoatlantoaxial (bones at the top of the neck) subluxation complex and a reduction in depressive symptoms in some people."

Another documented case study appearing in the 23 April 2008 issue of the *Journal of Vertebral Subluxation Research*, showed the improvement of a patient with major depression with chiropractic care. In this case study, a 46-year-old man suffering from his third bout of major depression presented himself for chiropractic care.

The author of the case study concluded: "This report details the life history and symptomology of a 46-year-old man suffering with major depression, the 11 months of chiropractic care, and the man's physical, social and mental response to correction of vertebral subluxations. This report supports the previous literature written regarding correction of vertebral subluxation and its positive effect on physical, mental and social wellbeing."

What we must all remember is this: everything in your body is controlled by the brain and the nerves that run from your brain to your body. In the case of depression, it is possible to have one part of the nervous system, called the sympathetic nervous system, on overdrive. We experience everything in life through our nervous system. If our nervous system is compromised, our life experience will be compromised – one more reason to seek safe and natural chiropractic care first, instead of only relying on medications.

The effectiveness of mainstream medications like antidepressants should not be undermined. Chiropractors do not suggest that someone suffering from depression should forgo mainstream medical treatments. However, we would strongly suggest complementing your medical treatment with chiropractic adjustments, working hand-in-hand with your health provider until such a time that your medication may no longer be necessary. I would not be able to count the number of patients over the years who have said to me a month or so into their care, "I don't need my anti-depressants any more. Since I started having my adjustments, I just feel so much better!" The magic of our innate intelligence *is* boundless.

Depression is expected to be the second largest killer after heart disease by 2020 and studies show it to be a contributing factor to fatal coronary disease. Sounds like a great reason to have you and your family checked for subluxations on a regular basis!

Another aspect of depression and anxiety is what is termed Panic Disorder. It is a disorder characterised by constant and sudden attacks of extreme fear and nervousness. The attacks are normally not connected to any particular situation and usually last for about 10 minutes. The cause of panic disorder is still unidentified, but it is believed that it is related with many physiological factors. It *can* happen to children, but the average age it usually occurs is around 25. It can also affect adults and seniors. According to recent studies, women are 2–3 times more prone to panic disorders.

What Are the Symptoms? Panic attacks include limited periods of severe symptoms; some of these may be:

- Difficulty breathing
- Light-headedness or faintness
- Tremors
- Trembling
- Too much perspiration
- Choking
- Abdominal pain and nausea
- Lack of feeling or tingling
- Chest pain
- Chills
- Necrophobia (fear of dying)
- Afraid of becoming crazy
- Fear of losing control

Most patients with undiagnosed panic disorder might feel they are dying. Usually, they immediately proceed to the emergency room or health centre because of a feeling they are having a heart attack. I once adjusted one of my patients literally on her way home from the hospital after experiencing a panic attack. She knew that she wasn't dying and her heart was ok, so she came in to see me. She was still sweating and hyperventilating and acting like a cat on a hot tin roof. I checked her spine for subluxations and found problems in her upper neck and around T6 (bra strap area). I adjusted her and as soon as I had completed the adjustment, she returned to her normal behaviour. It was instant, in this case, which amazed both her and I, and other patients who had witnessed her distress. In chiropractic, when we perform anterior adjustments of the thoracic spine, it can directly affect the function of the autonomic nervous system, bringing the body back into balance very quickly.

I have had many patients report similar changes – some not as rapid but, nevertheless, just as life-changing for that person. I look after a lovely man who comes in once a month with his wife for his regular check up. He was literally dragged in by his wife and daughter who hoped that I might be able to improve his depressive symptoms and stress levels. He had no physical symptoms at all, and wondered why he should see a chiropractor. A few short weeks into his care, I noticed a change in his demeanor which continued to improve as the weeks passed. I will never forget the time he shared with me that he was feeling so much better on the inside, and life didn't seem so hard anymore. I always look forward to seeing him and his wife now, as we enjoy a great laugh together.

Anxiety and depression frequently target any weak areas of the spine and can cause general muscular tension, headaches, migraine, neck and back pain. This pain can, in turn, aggravate the already present anxiety and depression in some individuals.

Chronic pain can cause severe anxiety and depressive symptoms over time. This can manifest itself in a decrease of social interaction and activity, as well as general feelings of remorse or sadness when dealing with ongoing pain, and a sense of hopelessness at the situation when relief has not been found. Studies have shown, however, that proper chiropractic treatment can greatly reduce not only the physical ailments, but the mental anguish that often accompanies them. Stress, anxiety and depression can be alleviated by successful chiropractic care.

If the source of pain is isolated and treated and the pain is relieved, one's general sense of mood will lift and there will be renewed invigoration for once difficult (but normally routine) tasks. Overall, the individual starts to feel better in every sense.

Another patient I currently look after had experienced neck pain for a few years, as well as depression, anxiety and bipolar symptoms. Upon examination, her C2 (second top vertebrae in her neck) was severely out of alignment. The first adjustment made a small change to her symptoms, but as the weeks passed she noticed not only her neck improving but also her internal world. Her life has changed so dramatically since we began treatment, even her sister popped in to let me know how wonderfully it has affected not only her sibling, but also the extended family. When the messages from the brain to the body are not getting through properly, the magnificence that lies within us cannot shine to its full potential, preventing the vital expression of life. How lucky I am to witness such miracles as a chiropractor.

For many years now, as well as adjusting patients I have also presented Wellbeing programs. These programs consist of workshops and also individual coaching sessions. The workshops cover nutrition, exercise, chiropractic, mind power, emotions and spiritual evolution. The coaching addresses the person's highest health priorities, whatever they may be. To my surprise, more than 80% of the participants suffered from depression and/or anxiety. Looking after the person on every level, as mentioned above, results in such profound changes in people's lives it is truly amazing.

We are funny creatures we humans. Sometimes we try to make it so complicated and get all frustrated when we don't understand everything.

Let's just keep it simple:

- Nourish your body with nutritious natural food.

- Exercise daily.

- Ensure your brain is communicating with your body without interference.

- Keep your thoughts positive – live your life from love, not fear.

- And walk the path laid before you this lifetime.

Told you it was easy!

CHAPTER 35

*"Common sense in an uncommon degree is
what the world calls wisdom."*

Samuel Taylor Coleridge

Those Legs
are Made
for Walking

By Bruce Whittingham

I remember Ellen coming into my office; she had been crying. Ellen was 12
years old and had been chosen to represent England in the European under
14's springboard diving championships in two weeks. She was experiencing
excruciating knee pain and had been to her doctor who had delivered the
crushing diagnosis of Osgood Schlaters disease (inflammation of the bump on
the front, upper part of the lower leg bone, causing pain and swelling below the
knee) which meant six weeks off her feet to let the swelling subside. As far as
Ellen was concerned this was as good as saying all that she had worked for was
over – she had been diving since she was eight years old and this was her first
chance to represent her country – and possibly her last!

So why come to a chiropractor for knee pain? Fortunately, I had been working with the team for over a year by then and they knew that I was good with headaches, wrist sprains and elbows – maybe I knew something about knees as well. What is interesting is that chiropractors see pain as a symptom, and symptoms only occur when the body is stressed beyond its ability to cope.

Pain is the body's warning sign (like the warning lights on the dashboard of a car) that if we repeat what we have done we will get more of the same – PAIN! A pretty good deterrent, helping to prevent further injury.

The problem with pain is that most people and doctors look at the site of pain and forget about the body around it. They will ice it, immobilise it, inject it, and even operate on it, but all too often this doesn't heal it!

Ellen's pain was coming from the insertion of her infra patella tendon tearing from its insertion into the tibia. This creates an acute inflammatory response which sends searing pain into the knee every time the quadriceps muscle is contracted. This makes it painful to walk, but excruciating to climb stairs, which springboard divers have to do for hours a day when training and competing.

The diagnosis was absolutely correct – tearing and acute inflammation on the tibial insertion of the patella ligament. But why on the right side only? Climbing stairs is a balanced activity and not every diver in her group had the same condition! In order to have tearing at this point, the quadriceps had to be hypertonic (i.e. have a high degree of tension). Looking at the whole limb we could see that her right foot was pronating (turning in), her knee was stressed medially (as with knocked knees), her pelvis was twisting and this was stressing the quadriceps.

> *The leg works as a kinematic chain – to take a step you need to move the bones of the foot, the ankle, the knee, the hip and the pelvis in a uniform movement. If one of these links is not moving as it should it puts stress on all the others.*

We worked on Ellen's quadriceps, adjusted her pelvis, hip, knee and foot and arranged for her to use orthotics to support her feet at all times (even at home and at the pool). Ellen made it to the European championships, she even scoured a personal best and a place in the top three – even though she felt a little self conscious walking backwards up the stairs to her dive platform during all her practice sessions.

When we have pain in the joints of our arms or legs, we soon learn just how much of an inconvenience this is, and often repetitive strain injuries of these joints can take years to settle because we find it impossible to live our lives without using the injured limbs, which just adds insult to injury and prevents healing from taking place. But again it is often the location of the pain that gets all the attention and treatment rather than the whole limb and ergonomics of the person's workplace or sporting activity associated with the repetitive nature of the stress.

Often a well delivered adjustment, which restores the correct movement through the whole limb and releases pressure, can dramatically improve the healing time.

But what of the silent subluxation – the subluxation that does not elicit any symptom or pain? We know how these can create degeneration of discs in the spine but what about the limbs? The limbs are so often neglected when looking at the subluxation pattern of an individual.

A subluxation pattern develops as the whole body has tried to compensate for imbalances and stress on a nerve or groups of nerves anywhere in the body.

Take a pebble in your shoe, for example. Now it doesn't have to be a big pebble to create an irritation to the foot, but you can still walk to the corner store and back with a pebble in your shoe. Your body just makes a few alterations to the way you distribute weight on the foot – by changing the angle of the pelvis, twisting the knee and even everting the foot (turning it outwards) if needed. If, however, you have to run a marathon with the pebble in your shoe, you will probably reach a point where the compensations you have had to make will result in symptoms because the strain on the body has exceeded its limits and it needs you to make some changes.

At this point of pain, it may be your knee that hurts, or your low back – but let's say it's a blister on the sole of your foot from the pebble rubbing the skin. You can choose to stop running and rest it in the hope the inflammation will settle, maybe a little cream or ointment might help. Now of course you think this is silly; just take the pebble out of your shoe (which is obvious in this case). But all too often we aren't dealing with a pebble – we are too busy looking at the twisted pelvis or sore knee and don't even think to look in the shoe!

As a chiropractor I see the body as a whole, all of the cells working in a coordinated harmony to create health and wellbeing whilst adapting to the stresses we are subjected to, or, in most cases, subject ourselves to every day. Subluxations of the extremities will cause interference of nocioceptors (nerves around the subluxated joint) which travel to the spinal cord and on to the cerebellum at the brain stem affecting the higher centres of the brain which control muscle tone, stress, balance etc. Dr Mark Charette refers to this nerve irritation as "internal noise" which the brain has to contend with 24 hours a day whilst the subluxation is present. The greater the number of subluxations, the more intensity will affect the volume of this noise – no wonder people get irritable and stressed, have difficulty concentrating, and sleep poorly.

Due to our repetitive work and recreational movements, we create repetitive stress around the joints in our arms and legs. This is why we so often hear terms like "frozen shoulder", "tennis elbow" and even "RSI" for repetitive strain injury. All too often these acute states can be prevented by screening the limbs for subluxation, correcting postural stresses by using ergonomic supports, and stretching on a regular basis – at the start and end of every day. Each day we are taking part in an endurance event, working for up to eight hours using the same muscle groups (even if it is sitting at a computer). Now most of us would not consider going for a long run without stretching, yet going to work does not get the same respect, even though our survival depends on it!

The most overlooked part of our anatomy though, has to be our feet! They are all the way down there, often covered and even called ugly. I am a self-confessed foot basher. From a young age I had what is commonly known as pancake feet – totally flat. This was of my own doing as I had run two marathons, at age 14 and 16, and being 181cm tall and weighing 95 kg I am not built for that event!

I went on to rupture both of my medial collateral knee ligaments, and I couldn't run more than 3 km without getting shin splints or knee pain. I tried orthotics off the shelf and even had casts made of my feet for custom orthotics, which helped the foot soreness and the shin splints but I still couldn't run past 3 km without knee pain. As the years progressed I found my feet would burn at the end of a long day and even my low back would stiffen up – not a good situation for a chiropractor having regular adjustments.

Eventually I realised that all I was being offered was support for the medial arch of my foot, where we actually have three arches. The mid-foot has a medial arch on the instep, which we all feel when we buy a new pair of joggers, a lateral arch on the outside edge of the foot, and a transverse arch in the middle, just forward of the other two arches. I found a company that could provide support for all three arches and now I can run 10 km without knee or shin pain and no longer have low back stiffness or burning feet.

The interesting thing is, when I began to support my patients' feet correctly, they actually held their adjustments better. A simple muscle test can be done to see if the arches of your feet are functioning well. Stand on one bare foot, raise the other knee so the thigh is at 90 degrees to the ground, and have someone test the strength of the raised leg by pushing the raised knee towards the ground. In over 90 per cent of patients I have tested, there is an easy-to-demonstrate weakness. The reason for this is that not only do the arches in the feet act as springs to absorb load as we walk or run, they also help provide stability for the body when we stand.

In fact, some studies show that by the age of 20, 80 per cent of us have dropped arches (often the outside/lateral arch and the anterior/transverse arches are the first to drop). The reason is our feet are designed to walk on sand, soil and clay, which our feet can grip and mould into. Instead, our feet are subjected to surfaces such as concrete, tiles and hardwood flooring with little support in our shoes, if we are even wearing anything on our feet. (Consider how many steps you take when you are at home. An active person can take as many as 10,000 steps per day.)

The irony is that most patients, having had a great adjustment, may be re-creating stress through their body with each step they take as they walk out of the room, due to poor arch support in their feet. So please ask your chiropractor to check your arches to make sure your feet are supporting your body optimally.

Extremities are an important part of the whole – look after them with chiropractic care.

CHAPTER 36

"The art of chiropractic is much more than an application of a technique or an introduction of a force. It is a melding of substance and being; of technical precision and heart centred connection. In the moment of the adjustment, two become one; a synergistic flow begins toward growth and evolution. The power and creativity of nature are unleashed, awakening us to the realization that the adjustment is alive and dynamically in motion."

Sue Brown, DC

Handling the Technique

By Monica Handa

So what is chiropractic technique all about and why would it interest you? Well, technique is described as "a mechanical skill in an art". So there you have it – the art part is chiropractic and the technique part is the manual administration of the adjustment, the why it is we do what we do. Lost already? Let me try to explain a bit more clearly. In chiropractic terms, almost all techniques are based on the delivery of a particular type of adjustment. An adjustment corrects a subluxation. There is a great diversity of techniques that chiropractors use, which is greatly beneficial to you the patient. It's about not one size fitting all, not trying to push round pegs into square holes, but a more bespoke approach to your health and healing potential. For example, a chiropractor would never use the same technique on a new born baby as they would on a rugby prop-forward! Technique is about modifying things so that you the patient get the best for you. If you are lucky enough to live in an area of the world where there is more than one chiropractor in your neighbourhood you may prefer to see one chiropractor over the other just because of the way they practise, including the type of technique they use.

Most chiropractors graduate from their college or university having learnt a few techniques and may even join a technique club at their place of study. The idea of a technique club is to become more proficient in delivering a particular style of adjustment. It is, after all, as described above, "a mechanical skill" and it takes time to become competent at a skill! Currently, most chiropractic institutions have at least one or two years where students practise the techniques of varying styles of adjustment on one another and also practise in a student out-patient clinic. These clinics are places where the student is let loose on the general public, under a great deal of supervision.

The techniques that are taught at college vary greatly from one institution to another. The chiropractor's choice of technique usually arises from patient need, the quest to be able to help more people, individual experiences and interest, and may even be down to the practice they joined when they first started to work. Almost all techniques will get the results you are looking for a majority of the time for example, let's say 90%. The desire to be able to help the 10% of people who don't respond to the original techniques applied is what usually drives chiropractors to seek out further methods of analysis; i.e. to help the few. In my experience, most chiropractors follow the procedures of a particular technique but almost always make minor alterations in the way they practise in order to suit the individual needs of the patient. After all, we are all unique and our bodies may respond differently to the same input/adjustment.

I still have conversations with patients, usually after their first adjustment, when they'll say something along the lines of "Who did you do that to first?"

The answer is that a chiropractor's first adjustment was probably done on another student. All students are tested to see whether they are capable before they are allowed to graduate. Usually they also have to have seen a minimum number of their own patients in the student out-patient clinic and delivered a minimum number of adjustments too, utilising a variety of techniques.

Most chiropractic techniques involve a method of analysis to discover where subluxations are present and then a method of dealing with the findings – a bit like a flow chart. The analysis could be reductionist, looking at the symptoms in isolation, or it could be wholistic, looking at the presenting symptoms as they fit in with the whole of you. At the end of the day, as has already been described elsewhere in this book, the objective of any chiropractic technique is to simply remove or reduce nerve interference. This allows the brain and the body to communicate with one another as efficiently as possible so allowing the body to function and heal to the best of its ability – allowing you to reach your optimum potential.

Different ideas as to the primary causes of subluxations can be one way of understanding why there is a wide range of techniques as well as different ideas as to the solutions. Overall, there are more similarities than differences, but each technique has its own particular place in the broad realm of everyday practice. The more prominent adjusting techniques taught at chiropractic colleges are Diversified, Thompson, Activator, Gonstead, Sacro Occipital Technique, Logan Basic and Toggle Recoil. As time goes by, more and more techniques continue to evolve. What follows below is a brief description of more commonly known chiropractic techniques. Although chiropractors focus primarily on the spine, there are also special techniques used to adjust other areas of the body, such as the shoulders, ribs, elbows, wrists and hands, knees, ankles and feet.

Diversified Technique

Diversified is the most known and practised of all chiropractic techniques.[1]

It was developed by the founder of chiropractic, DD Palmer, and is taught in all chiropractic colleges. This is a purely manual, hands-on approach and no instruments are used during the adjustments. The analysis of your concerns comes from taking case histories, sometimes x-rays, and feeling the individual joints that are subluxated. You may hear a popping noise when adjustments are delivered as this technique concentrates on restoration to normal biomechanical function, and correction of subluxation. In addition, Diversified techniques have been used to adjust extremity joints, allowing for beneficial applications in treating sports injuries and other injuries.

Thompson Technique

Chiropractor Dr J Clay Thompson, the originator of this technique, produced a special type of bench in the late 1950s, the original Thompson point terminal bench, which had sections in it that would drop and give way with only a small amount of additional force. This was in order to enhance the force applied to the area being adjusted. There are now many benches (known as "drop piece tables") that have similar mechanisms. The chiropractor pushes on a particular part of your body in order to make the bench move under you, thus moving the joint. Most of the spinal adjusting utilising the Thompson Technique has the patient lying prone (face down). The thrusts that are applied to the spine take into account the inherent design of the spine and the way in which the joints line up.

Dr Derefield added another dimension to the Thompson technique. He noted adjusting patients with identical analyses did not produce identical results. So the Derefield-Thompson technique relies upon a very accurate leg length analysis and balancing out of the legs may be achieved by turning the head in a particular direction.[2]

Activator Methods

Activator Methods chiropractic technique was developed by chiropractors

Warren Lee and Arlan Fuhr. Initially, the doctors used thumb thrusts, delivered at rapid rates of speed generated by elbow movement. They developed the "Activator" instrument to avoid injuries to doctors (resulting from the thumb thrusts) and to ensure consistency from one adjustment to the next. Activator technique utilises an activator, which is a small hand-held spring loaded instrument that delivers a thrust upon use and can be set to deliver force ranging from nine to 33 pounds per square inch. A leg test is used to check for the presence of subluxations and these tests can be used to check adjustment effectiveness afterwards. The emphasis is on the specific speed and line of drive (the direction in which the activator is positioned), to accomplish effective reduction of subluxations within the body, rather than any degree of force. Activator Methods adjustments can also be used on extremity joints. The Activator Methods technique comes about from a mixture of several other chiropractic techniques including Derefield-Thompson and Logan Basic.[3,4]

Gonstead Technique

Dr Clarence Gonstead developed the Gonstead technique using principles based upon engineering models. He practised for 51 years, gaining empirical data during that time to further develop his technique. The premise behind the technique is based upon the following: the body's foundation is formed by the pelvic girdle. When this bony structure (consisting of hip bones) and the lower bones of the back are level, there will be maximum balance and stability in the spinal column. When the pelvic girdle or any of the vertebrae (bones making up the spinal column) become tilted or rotated out of their proper position, dramatic changes may occur in the body.

The Gonstead technique utilises five criteria to detect the presence of the vertebral subluxation complex. They are: observation (of posture and movement), instrumentation (an instrument is used to check for uneven distributions of heat along the spine), static palpation (feeling the spine in a stationary position), motion palpation (feeling the spine whilst moving and bending), and x-ray analysis (taken of the full spine in the upright position to evaluate posture, joint and disc integrity and misaligned vertebrae, and to check for fractures or pathology).

After completing the above analysis, the chiropractor is ready to deliver any necessary adjustments. The focus of the Gonstead adjustment is to be as specific, precise and accurate as possible, addressing only the areas of subluxation. Great care is taken to ensure a bio-mechanically correct position and precise thrust to provide the most accurate and painless adjustment possible.[5]

Sacro Occipital Technique

Sacro Occipital Technique (SOT) was developed by Dr Bertrand De Jarnette, a wealthy former engineer who used much of his fortune funding research on why chiropractic works. De Jarnette concluded that structural changes affecting the dura can affect any area of the spine. The dura covers the entire central nervous system (the brain and the spinal cord). De Jarnette based his conclusions in part on the fact that adjusting one segment of the spine may bring about a change in another area of the spine.

Additionally, De Jarnette was interested in research showing that cranial bones move and theorised that structural changes of the cranial bones could affect the movement of cerebrospinal fluid (fluid surrounding the brain and spinal cord). Thus, SOT addresses positioning of the cranial bones, using a method known as craniopathy.

SOT gets its name because it recognises, and uses, the relationship between the sacrum (base of the spine) and the occiput (base of the skull) as a key to proper body function. Typically, an SOT chiropractor uses a simple, non-force method of adjusting your spine, pelvis and cranium.

SOT also uses wedge shaped blocks for addressing pelvic subluxations to allow the body to seek its correct alignment and balance. These are placed under the pelvis with the patient lying face up. The goal is to normalise joint positions on both sides of the spine simultaneously.

There are many combinations of block positions used, and these are determined by tests that precede each adjustment. SOT integrates with other chiropractic systems, allowing for use of a variety of techniques within the SOT system. Practitioners also often provide nutritional counselling to patients.[6,7]

Logan Basic

Logan Basic was developed by chiropractor HB Logan and is one of the lowest-force adjustive techniques. The technique is based on light, sustained force exerted against a specific contact point on the sacrum at the base of the spine. Additional contacts at various points in the spine, or along specific muscles, can also be used. The technique uses the muscular structure surrounding the sacrum as a lever system for balancing the entire structure of the spine.

Integral to use of Logan Basic Technique is the Logan System of Body Mechanics, Dr Logan's system of calculating compensatory mechanisms, which occur as a result of postural distortions, and correction of those distortions.[8]

Cox Technique

Cox Technique founder Dr Cox explains his technique (aka Flexion-Distraction) as a marriage of chiropractic principles with osteopathic principles. Cox Flexion-Distraction is a gentle, non-force adjusting procedure that works with the body's natural design to aid it in healing. Dr Cox developed and enhanced a special table, a Flexion-Distraction table, to be used in conjunction with a distractive force (supplied with the contact hand). Distracting the spine and then flexing it (using table motion) can resolve pain from joint and disc problems painlessly. The table is designed to restore normal ranges of movement to the neck, mid back and lower back. Additional goals of the Flexion-Distraction adjustment include transfer of nutrients into the spinal disc, decreasing pressures between the discs and decompressing inflamed/compressed spinal nerve roots. Therefore it is a powerfully effective, conservative approach to low back and leg pain, and an alternative to explore before seeking surgery.[9]

Chiropractic Biophysics

In December 1980, Chiropractic BioPhysics® (or CBP®) Technique, was originally named by chiropractors Dr Donald Harrison, Dr Deanne Harrison, and Dr Daniel Murphy for *"physics applied to biology in chiropractic"*. Since that time, Drs Donald and Deed Harrison, (along with a number of other contributors) have written seven CBP text books and published more than 130 scientific studies investigating different aspects of CBP. Thus, today, CBP Technique is one of the foremost investigated techniques in chiropractic and both Dr Don and Dr Deed are among the leaders in the profession's researchers.

CBP Technique emphasizes optimal posture and spinal alignment as the primary goals of chiropractic care while simultaneously documenting improvements in pain and functional based outcomes. The uniqueness of CBP treatment is in the structural rehabilitation of the spine and posture. So CBP technique goes beyond a reduction in symptoms and can be likened to orthodontics for the spine. X-rays must be taken in order to achieve the changes in alignment, which are achieved with postural corrective adjustments, postural corrective exercises and postural corrective traction. In general, the goals of CBP care are: normal front and side view postures; normal spinal alignment from the front and side views; and normal function and improvements in health and symptoms.[10]

Pierce-Stillwagon Technique

Chiropractors Glenn Stillwagon and Vern Pierce developed this technique in 1963. The technique is a system of analysing and adjusting the spine that combines previously understood concepts with a very simplified, logical and effective procedure to correct subluxations. This full spine technique requires the use of a "hi-lo table" with pelvic drop pieces and cervical pads. It uses x-ray analysis, instrumentation (thermography, which measures skin temperature) and other physical findings to produce a reproducible care plan for patients. The adjustment is given by hand in a high speed, low-force manner.[11]

Motion Analysis (Palpation)

This technique, in which the practitioner's hands are used to feel the motion of specific segments of the spine and extremities during movement, was developed by Henri Gillet, a Belgian chiropractor. Since its introduction in the early 1980s it has quickly gained acceptance as a standard diagnostic tool for the chiropractic profession. Motion palpation is now taught in chiropractic colleges throughout the world. Motion Analysis was created as a system of spinal analysis that permits an easy examination of the spine, both in pinpointing the different subluxations and in determining their types. This system also serves in determining direction and force of adjustment. It was found that subluxations can be classed according to the degree of restriction of mobility. It was also found that correction of the subluxation usually has a spontaneous correcting effect on smaller fixations. In addition, when the key subluxation in any series is discovered and corrected, there was found to be a series of fixations which usually occured together and disappeared together.[12]

Applied Kinesiology

In 1964, chiropractor George Goodhart made an observation that when he treated a weak muscle, its strength could be improved. The technique has now evolved and is used as a form of diagnosis to examine how a person's body is functioning by testing the strength of muscles. When a muscle test determines a muscle is weak, the practitioner attempts to find out why. Various therapies can be used to strengthen the muscles including adjustments, soft tissue work, cranial work and nutritional approaches, to name but a few. In some cases, the examiner may test for environmental or food sensitivities by using a previously strong muscle to find what weakens it. There are many other techniques that use Applied Kinesiology, e.g. Neural Organizational Therapy (NOT) and Neuro Emotional Technique (NET).[13]

Upper Cervical (neck) Techniques

There are a number of techniques that focus on adjusting just the joints of the upper neck, i.e. the occiput (skull), atlas (first vertebra) and the axis (second vertebra). They all involve a method of x-ray analysis to assess the positions of the atlas and the axis. The adjustments are often followed up by another x-ray to check for the effectiveness of the adjustment and the level of correction achieved. The adjustment can be administered using the hands or by using an adjusting instrument. The hand-delivered adjustment involves a light contact and a shallow thrust. The contact point, the pisiform (a small bone on the inside corner of your hand), usually travels less than 3/16" (approx 6 mm) during the thrust. Many chiropractors utilize a hand-held electrically powered instrument to deliver a very quick and shallow thrust, or various forms of table-mounted instruments. Atlas specific technique was founded by Wernsing in the 1930s and derivative techniques include Grostic, Nucca, Pettibon, Orthospinology, Hole-In-One and Atlas Orthogonal.[14,15,16,17,18]

Other Techniques

There are a plethora of other techniques and the following take a look at the whole spine – Advanced Biostructural Correction, Bio-Geometric Integration, Cerebrospinal Fluid Technique (CSFT), Directional Non-Force Technique (DNFT), Network Spinal Analysis, Matrix Repatterning, Bio Energetic Synchronization Technique, and the list goes on and on.

Chirodontics is a specialist technique that focuses on jaw problems, headaches and cranio-facial pain syndromes.

Many chiropractors include some sort of 'soft tissue work' as an adjunct to their primary choice of technique. This is where the chiropractor (or someone else in the office) works on muscles and ligaments. Common techniques used for this purpose include Nimmo, Graston, Trigger Point Therapy and various types of massage.

Other commonly practised techniques include nutritional therapy, exercise, rehabilitation and the prescription of orthotics. All of these approaches add to the chiropractors "bag of tricks", in order to help you the patient reach a healthier state.

And finally, please do remember that different techniques take varying amounts of time to administer.

It's not how long it takes for the chiropractor to perform the adjustment(s) that matters, but the effect it will have on your body.

CHAPTER 37

"The significant problems we face cannot be solved at the same level of thinking we were at when we created them."

Albert Einstein

Ever been told to "Just live with it"?

It's Never Too Late, No Matter How Old You Are

By Cathy Turnell

I f you have experienced a gradual deterioration in your ability to participate in a more active lifestyle into your retirement years, or if you are one of the older generation who has one or more debilitating health conditions, chiropractic is able to help.

Chiropractors are used to seeing people who have a variety of complaints while they are being co-managed with general medicine, and one of the most common problems chiropractors see, particularly in middle-aged or elderly people, is osteoarthritis, also known as spinal or joint decay or, more commonly, wear and tear. Osteoarthritis is characterised by decreased movement in the spinal or extremity joints, and to begin with, is not always accompanied by pain. The decrease in joint movement is followed by muscle, ligament and bone remodelling resulting in restricted joint movement and, in its end stage, complete fusion of the joints. Osteoarthritis can result in reduced physical mobility, pain, mood changes, and reduced quality of life.

Even though it's diagnosed in young people, in general, conventional medicine views osteoarthritis as a consequence of aging and it is considered to be an inevitable factor in growing old. Although osteoarthritis leads to discomfort and a poor quality of life, the process in itself is not directly life threatening. This means that the symptoms are normally managed first with drugs such as anti-inflammatories, anti-depressants with muscle-relaxant side effects, and tranquilisers or analgesics in extreme cases. People are often referred to a physiotherapist for rehabilitation. In the end stages of osteoarthritis the last option may be surgery to replace worn out joints.

Chiropractors, on the other hand, view osteoarthritis as a side effect of a lack of proper maintenance of the joints. Over the years, the joints begin to deteriorate after being exposed to a variety of lifestyle stressors such as chronic dehydration, a deficiency of vital nutrients, and the major contributor – a lack of daily, regular spinal movement.

If the body is intelligent how does osteoarthritis develop?

The body is controlled moment to moment by a force called innate intelligence, so, considering that osteoarthritis is a source of suffering that reduces our ability to do the things in life that we love as we get older, how can chiropractors view osteoarthritis as an intelligent adaptation for the body to develop? To answer this question we need to ask ourselves, in the context of the *survival* of the whole body, what the spine and the spinal joints are designed to do, and what the body will choose to do if it is exposed to chronic deficiencies and toxicities.

The spine is primarily designed to protect the delicate spinal cord and the nerves exiting the spine. The spinal joints are also designed to allow us to move freely all day every day. Our ancestors would have been moving, stretching, reaching, lifting and hauling every day to acquire food and shelter just to survive, so any hunter-gatherers that were sedentary died out and active hunter-gatherers took precedence.[3] In these conditions, movement and physical activity was needed simply to survive, and as a consequence of the activity levels of our ancestors, the human brain has become dependent on movement signals from the body in order to thrive[2]; or put another way, movement is now like a nutrient for proper brain function. The amount of physical movement, and especially stretching and challenging the spine throughout its physical range of motion, has dramatically reduced as we have become more industrialised and therefore more sedentary in our pursuits. Unfortunately, this reduction in our daily movement is not so compatible with the degree of activity the human body needs to thrive.

So what happens when we sit for several hours at a time, not stretching or moving the spine? How does the brain interpret this? Well, all joints, including the spine, are designed to move *all the time*. Therefore the brain is expecting movement information to be feeding back to it from the joints *all the time*. This feedback of movement information is called "proprioception". Proprioception signals are what maintain healthy joints and, more importantly, contribute to a healthy nervous system. If a joint is not moved for as little as 45–60 minutes, the amount of proprioception (healthy nerve signals) to the brain is reduced.[2] When this occurs, the brain intelligently reasons that if a joint (designed to move remember!) stops moving then some kind of injury must have occurred to the joint. If an injury has taken place then some healing and repair needs to begin. So the brain intelligently activates the inflammatory cycle in and around the stationary joints. This sparks the start of scar tissue deposition in the joints, to try and repair the area. This deposition is the start of spinal decay.[8,9]

Most of us can quickly reverse this effect by stretching and moving the body to create proprioception signals and maintain the movement of the joints. However, a lack of movement is not the whole story. If the body is continually exposed to other physical, chemical and emotional stressors, then this will also predispose the body to developing spinal decay.

Aside from movement, the joints require the surrounding fluid (called synovial fluid) to lubricate and facilitate joint movement. This fluid is comprised largely of water and protein. Most of us fail to meet our daily water requirements for *health* (which is more than the requirement for only survival) and, as a result, expose the body to chronic low levels of hydration over many years. Once again we must reflect on what choices the innate intelligence will make if it is chronically restricted to a basic requirement for health. Medicine views a dry mouth as a sign of dehydration. According to Dr Batmanghelidj, author of *Your Body's Many Cries For Water*[1], when your mouth is dry, your body is indicating that your dehydration level is extreme. This physical sign is the "last outward sign of extreme dehydration. The damage occurs at a level of persistent dehydration that does not necessarily demonstrate a dry mouth signal".

This means that when we continually choose fluids other than water to quench our thirst (tea, coffee, fruit juice or fizzy drinks) the innate intelligence begins to shut down our feelings of thirst. Why? Because the stomach is detecting that a volume of fluid has been taken in. But, the body is still actually suffering dehydration so after this behaviour is repeated over time, it doesn't bother activating thirst signals, the innate intelligence starts to increase our feelings of hunger. Why? *In order to get some water from the fruit and vegetables we should be eating.* Sadly though, what we generally eat nowadays when we are pushed for time in our busy lives, families and work schedules is largely dehydrated convenience food that does not contain substantial levels of water for the body to use. We need *water* for hydration.

When the body is put into a situation where its supply of this basic requirement for health is limited, it begins to ration the supply of water to different parts of the body, favouring the tissues of the vital organs over others. The tissues that are expendable, i.e. those you can survive (but not thrive) with when they're not working optimally, are the muscles, joints and ligaments. So in the situation where movement is depleted, it is difficult for the body to maintain healthy joints, which is then compounded by a lack of water and other nutrient components that allow the joints to move freely.

We all know the feeling after a deep sleep: the stiffness and soreness in the spine after hours lying down, and then how good a luxurious stretch feels. Stretching the spine bombards the brain with proprioceptive stimulation and you can immediately feel the difference in your body and in your levels of alertness afterwards. The stiffness we feel in the morning after a night lying in bed, or following a long car journey, signifies the start of spinal decay.

The good news is that you can take control of the situation and prevent the condition known as osteoarthritis from worsening, improve it, and even stop it from happening in the first place! How? The most basic requirements for spinal health are movement and water. Therefore, start regular spinal movement every day and throughout the day with simple spinal stretches. The longer you are sitting or performing the same activity, the more you need to be stretching the spine. Ensure that you are properly hydrated: drink 2 to 2.5 litres of fresh, clean water every day.

How can chiropractic help?

So how can being adjusted by a chiropractor help someone who has had a lifetime of stressors and the resulting spinal decay is moderate to severe? According to Wolff's law, if there is normal movement between two joint surfaces, even after some degeneration has begun, then those joints can repair and remodel into healthy functioning joints once more.[5,7] Before the repair can start however, it is necessary to remove any interference in the nerve signals to the muscles controlling the joints.[6] Chiropractic works with the body by removing the nerve interference. A healthy nervous system will allow the muscles to coordinate the movement of the joints more efficiently. The degree of recovery that can be achieved is determined by the level of spinal decay to begin with, as well as the enthusiasm of the person to make changes to their daily lifestyle habits.

Sheila's story

There have been some truly astonishing improvements in osteoarthritis in people receiving chiropractic care. Sheila had suffered an injury to her left knee. Unfortunately, the injury never properly healed and this left her with constant pain in her leg and back. As a consequence of her reduced levels of activity, Sheila had seen a dramatic deterioration in her quality of life because of the wear and tear that had developed in her joints. What follows is Sheila's chiropractic experience and how her life has been transformed by receiving chiropractic care.

Sheila was someone who arrived in a chiropractic practice as a last resort after a medical doctor told her to "just live with it". At 59 years of age, Sheila could not walk for any length of time without being in great pain. The start of the deterioration in her mobility had begun four years previously after a nasty fall in the street. Tests at the time showed no gross joint damage or fracture to the knee but her ability to walk or squat without stiffness or severe pain never went away. Since the accident, Sheila had put on a lot of weight as her physical activity levels had reduced considerably and on her first visit to the chiropractor she expressed how she was thoroughly disgruntled with the state of her body, that she wanted more quality from life and that her knee and back pain was stopping her.

After examining Shelia, the chiropractor explained that her spine was "subluxated", which was stopping her nervous system from communicating properly with her body. If this could be restored then perhaps she could walk more easily.

After two months of chiropractic care, Sheila was shocked and surprised by the improvements in her mobility. She was so confident in how her body was recovering that she decided to get a new puppy. This was a very big decision as she had given up hope of ever being fit enough again to look after a dog. Sheila felt that her walking had improved so much that she would be able to keep up with the physical commitment that looking after a dog required and that having the dog to walk daily would also keep her exercising regularly. However, it wasn't all uphill improvement. After about three months her knee became very inflamed again after the dog barrelled into her left leg when she was out walking. Though unhappy with this setback, Shelia was positive that if she could improve after four years of agony, she could get over this setback as well; and in a few months she did.

It is nearly three years since Sheila's first chiropractic adjustment. She still comes in to have her spine checked every month and says how she wishes she had started chiropractic care years ago.

Although Sheila was not in an age range we would class as "elderly", the incapacity she experienced was similar to that of an older person. While Sheila's experience with chiropractic is by no means an isolated case (though her infectious enthusiasm did stand out!) what people like her can teach us is that there is no-one who is beyond the help of chiropractic. Even if you have been written off and tried many forms of care as Sheila had, there is always hope – however small or large your health goal is or whatever your stage of sickness or health. If you want to make a transformation in your state of health, chiropractic can help you.

Biographies

Sarah Farrant

Sarah Farrant DC, B Sci, Grad Dip Psych, B Phys Ed, is an Amazon #1
International Best Seller, global selling and award-winning author of
The Vital Truth®, international speaker, mother of three and a vitalistic systems
and marketing mentor who was named in 2008 "One of The Most Influential
Chiropractors 40 Years And Under" by Today's Lifestyle Magazine.

Known to many as the "Mother of Vitalism" Dr Sarah has an unmatched
ability to take a business and vitalize it into gold by maximizing every
opportunity. Her unique approach to systems, marketing and the use of
vitalistic language is transforming lay people, practice members, practices
and business owners around the globe. Dr Sarah's ability and her unwavering
trust has enabled her to become one of today's most sort after, successful and
influential female entrepreneurs. She is the founder and CEO of Vital Practice
Essentials and is committed to empowering professionals around the world to
start and grow their own business from a vitalistic perspective.

www.DrSarahFarrant.com

Rosemary Folker

Rosemary Folker BA(Hons) Norwich UK, who was born in Old Windsor in Buckinghamshire UK, had quite an unusual childhood in that she lived most of her young life on a boat.

She has been involved in Chiropractic her whole life (her grandfather was one of the first chiropractors to practice in the UK in 1932) and, upon marrying, supported her husband through chiropractic college. As a mature student with three children, she gained a first class honours degree in philosophy and sociology from the University of East Anglia in 1997 (one of only a handful of firsts ever awarded in that subject).

Since then, Rosemary has devoted her time to overseeing her husband's busy practices in Norwich and Holt in Norfolk, also spending a couple of years in Australia, running a practice in Melbourne. With 27 years experience under her belt, she does her utmost to ensure patient's expectations are not just met, but exceeded.

Passionate about the profession and its future direction, Rosemary was one of the people to suggest, and actively participate in, the forming of the first association (the United Chiropractic Association) in the UK to give a voice to chiropractors practising in a wellness model.

E: rosemary@norwichchiropractic.co.uk
www.norwichchiropractic.co.uk

Jennifer Layton B.Sc., Grad. Dip. Chiro. is a chiropractor in Lindfield, Sussex in the UK. An Australian, she first established her practice in Brisbane, Australia after graduating from Sydney University and Sydney College of Chiropractic.

Subsequently, Jennifer taught Chiropractic at Macquarie University for five years. However, her enthusiasm for travel and adventure took hold and she made the move to the UK and settled in Sussex from where she can continue to see the other side of the world. She enjoys skiing and tennis, and taking her children, Sebastian and Saskia, on escapades through Europe, and has won awards for her chocolate cakes.

Jennifer has done postgraduate studies in paediatrics and acupuncture, and is passionate about Chiropractic and how it can help people of all ages.

www.lindfieldchiro.co.uk

Paula Moore

Paula J Moore BA, BSc, MSc (Chiropractic), Fellow (CBP) was born in Toronto, Canada in 1967. Her kindergarten teacher described her as a dreamer, and she had her first successful business by the age of nine, selling used golf balls.

Her first degree was in Mathematics, graduating in 1990. Her introduction to Chiropractic came in her early twenties. She had been suffering from headaches for five years when she visited a chiropractor who introduced her to the magic of chiropractic. Her headaches resolved rapidly. So inspired was she by this natural approach to health, that she moved to England to complete two further degrees and qualified as a chiropractor in 2001. Paula's entire family now enjoy the benefits of chiropractic care.

Paula is passionate about good, healthy posture and has undertaken extensive post-graduate training in CBP (Clinical Biomechanics of Posture). She loves working with children and believes that those who have the benefit of chiropractic care have a head start in life. She also holds a post-graduate diploma in Paediatric Chiropractics.

When not giving chiropractic adjustments or attending courses, Paula may be found doing a spot of media, collecting driftwood, writing her blog or enjoying her morning exercise routine.

---

www.womenclimbingtrees.com

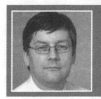

Neil Folker DC Norwich UK, graduated from Anglo-European College of Chiropractic in 1982, having received the award for Best Academic Record. He originally set up practice in Aylesbury, Buckinghamshire whilst also working at an established busy practice in Reading. In 1985, he and his wife and family moved to Norwich in Norfolk, where he runs a thriving practice offering wellness care to patients of all ages.

In 2003, Neil took the unusual step of relocating to Melbourne, Australia for a couple of years running a practice in one of the suburbs. He says it was certainly an experience running three practices on opposite sides of the world! Returning in 2005, he moved his Norwich practice into a 16th century building, originally the palace of the Bishop of Norwich.

With a keen interest in personal development and behavioural change, Neil believes that people are more likely to make beneficial changes to their health and lifestyle if they are well informed and supported throughout their care. He has travelled the globe studying with the likes of Deepak Chopra and Tony Robbins.

He was one of the founder members of the United Chiropractic Association and served as the Association's president for the first three years.

E: drneil@norwichchiropractic.co.uk
www.norwichchiropractic.co.uk
www.drneilfolker.com

Alan Scott BSc (Chiro) D.C. graduated from the Anglo-European College of Chiropractic (AECC) in 1993 and has been working in Newcastle upon Tyne in the North East of England since then. He has had his own practice in Gosforth for more than fifteen years, initially working with associates but now he prefers to work alone.

Since graduating, Alan has been interested in the diversity of techniques and approaches within the profession. He has studied Sacro-Occipital Technique for many years and more recently has converted his practice to Activator Method, which uses an adjusting instrument (an Activator).

Having had a diving injury to his neck as a child and suffering with headaches and growing pains, Alan is only too aware of what can happen when a spine is damaged.

As a chiropractor his goal is simple – to make people better and help them prevent problems in the future.

Alan has two beautiful children, Zak and Jasmine, who have each had chiropractic care since soon after birth and get adjusted regularly.

Shield Chiropractic
15 Princes Road Brunton Park, Gosforth
Newcastle upon Tyne, NE3 5TT

P: 0191 217 0387
E: info@shieldchiro.co.uk
www.shieldchiro.co.uk

I am **Anna Kurz Rogers** and I am 44 years old. I am married to a wonderful loving husband and we have four children aged 21, 18, 12 and 4 (three sons and one daughter).

I grew up on the Mornington Peninsula in Victoria, Australia and had a wonderful childhood spending weekends on the beach sailing and in later years windsurfing.

My husband and I moved to the Sunshine Coast in Queensland 20 years ago and have raised our children there in a sunny healthy lifestyle. A year after arriving I met my best friend Cyndi O'Meara and her husband Howard who showed me a wonderful healthy way of living, and my family and I have never looked back. Cyndi and I are so close and share everything – I am so lucky and fortunate to have her in my life.

We now live in the Sunshine Coast hinterland on an organic 50-acre hobby farm with our horses, pet sheep and chickens. My husband and I run our own business, our two eldest children have left home and we are raising the young boys in a beautiful environment.

Life could not be better …

Linda Power

Linda B Power DC, Dip SOTOA is one of the most experienced and highest qualified chiropractors in Australia with an expertise in safe and effective chiropractic health care for new born (only minutes old) to 90 plus, and a proven track record with patients still healthy and happy after maintaining care for over 30 years.

She graduated with a Doctor of Chiropractic magna cum laude from Palmer College of Chiropractic in 1976 and has done the Carrick neurology course. She has not only Basic and Advanced certification in Sacro-Occipital Technique (SOT) , but also Craniopath, and Diplomat in same, and was awarded a Life Membership by the Sacro Occipital Technique Organisation of Australasia in 2009 – the highest honour given out by this organisation. She is a past president of SOTOA and was nominated for *Who's Who* of Australia.

She has run successful practices for 35 years, taught Chiropractic to chiropractors and students since 1985, and mentored many new chiropractors who have gone on to become highly successful in their own businesses. Currently she maintains two wholistic chiropractic health care practices in Australia – one on the Sunshine Coast in Queensland and one in Woollahra, Sydney.

As a proud mother of two children and wife of a wonderful man, she is passionate about her practice and her patients.

Sunshine Coast:

E: drlinda@powerofhealth.com.au
P: +61 (0)7 5448 9544

Sydney:

E: drlpower1@bigpond.com
P: +61 (0)2 9389 3755

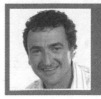

Wayne Whittingham

Wayne Whittingham DC, FCC, PhD – I was fortunate enough to be born into a chiropractic family – both my brother and sister are also practising chiropractors, one in Australia and one in Sweden. I graduated from RMIT in Australia, where I continued with my studies to do my doctorate. I lectured at RMIT and conducted a clinical trial on headaches for five years which culminated in achieving my PhD, and I have continued to have a keen interest in chiropractic care as a treatment for headaches. I then returned to the UK to join the family practice in Plymouth.

I have published in peer review journals, represented the profession on national radio and TV, and was given the award for clinical excellence by the International Chiropractic Association in 1992. I was nominated for the Who's Who in health care and medicine in 1995.

Currently I work in an open room wellness practice with three associates. I am also the Provisional Regional Trainer and tutor for the College of Chiropractors, which I have enjoyed for the past 10 years. I enjoy inspiring and motivating new graduates to become chiropractors.

I am married to Tracey and have two daughters, Bonnie and Lilly, two sons, Isaac and Alex, and one step-daughter, Keira, who between them keep me busy in my free time.

Plymouth Chiropractic Clinic
152 Mannamead Road Hartley,
Plymouth PL3 5QL

P: (01752) 770131
E: Waynecw67@hotmail.co.uk
www.plymouthchiropractic.com

John Swatland

John Swatland B.App.Sc.(Chiro) – I was eight years old when I was inspired to become a chiropractor after a series of life-changing adjustments by Dr Ralph De Conte in Adelaide, Australia. After graduating from what is now RMIT University, Melbourne, in 1984, I began private practice in Adelaide. With Palmer graduate Dr Paul Sykes as my mentor, I spent three years absorbing the philosophy of chiropractic that lives in me and drives me still today.

After extended travels in Europe and locums in the UK, I practised in Guildford, Surrey for just over three years. Then followed nearly six years of locum work in England, both Irelands and Australia, before settling into practice in south east Queensland with my young family. I wanted to see the world and also be skilled and confident in practising my craft in any setting, anywhere.

With fellow graduate Lawson Heath, I have built a thriving practice that has a focus on families and whole-person, wellness chiropractic. I especially enjoy my regular patient workshops where we explore a wide variety of healing topics from chiropractic and wellness philosophy to breathing techniques, meditation and healing and the mind (of course!).

Logan Hyperdome Chiropractic Centre
Unit 3, Logan Place, 3 Mandew St,
Shailer Park, Qld 4128

P: +61 (0)7 3801 5288
www.hyperdomechiro.com.au

Cyndi O'Meara BSc (Nutrition) – One serving from Australia's most provocative nutritionist, speaker and author will change lives! People can't get enough of Cyndi's O'Meara's recipe for a better life.

Individuals from neutral to all shades of green simply love the facts she dishes up – Diet Busters like "butter is best", "you don't need to diet" and "yes, you can eat choc chip cookies" which sit comfortably with "losing weight in 21 days", "beating Alzheimer's", "never needing antibiotics" and "staying at a healthy weight for life".

Flavour of the month every month, the talks that Cyndi presents tantalise, tempt and leave everyone satisfied. But it isn't just food to convert the fat and flabby. Cyndi brings a powerful "change your habits change your life" message that people at all ages and all stages of life are hungry to hear.

By offering palatable, easy directions for combating many contemporary ills – obesity, depression, heart disease and diabetes, drug dependence and exhaustion, stress and dysfunction – Cyndi wows the audience every time. Absolutely authentic and original, endearing, funny, inspirational, sincere and very entertaining, this unconventional nutritionist gives her audience exactly what they need.

Email **enquiries@changinghabits.com.au** for a detailed speaker profile or to enquire about Cyndi's availability for your next big event.

www.changinghabits.com.au

Alan Brown

Alan Brown, who is the father of three children, has been a practising chiropractor for more than 15 years.

His experience in a "wellbeing" culture started at the age of four after suffering for two years with chronic asthma which was not responding to conventional treatments. His mother explored a large range of alternative health professionals including chiropractors, naturopaths, osteopaths (including Tom Bowen, the originator of Bowen therapy). Not only did the symptoms of asthma resolve as a result of chiropractic care, but there was a tremendous change in his health generally. His family was brought up under very strong holistic health principles, which brought them closer as a family and healthier as individuals.

Drawing on his family experience, Alan now uses an eclectic approach with common sense chiropractic principles and enjoys helping families create health and wellbeing. He has worked across Australia and in the UK (as part of the oldest clinic in Scotland). Alan now runs a successful family practice in North Brisbane which takes care of a large proportion of the local area's expecting mums and children. He is passionate about family health and believes that the right approach can not only help illness but bring harmony, and ensure everyone gets the best out of family life.

Windsor Chiropractic Centre
65 Eildon Road,
Windsor Qld 4030

P: +61 (0)7 3357 3366
E: mail@windsorchiro.com www.
windsorchiro.com

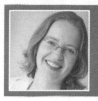

Kathy Knight B.MedSci, M.Chiro Webster Certified runs Universal Chiropractic, in Canberra, Australia. Her first experience of chiropractic care came as a child when she couldn't walk, following a fall while chasing her cat. Further experiences followed after spectacular sporting moments on the ski-slopes.

Kathy was born and raised in Canberra but left at 18 to begin her journey towards becoming a chiropractor. She began a Medical Science degree at the University of Sydney and discovered a passion for chiropractic, so furthered her studies by undertaking a Master in Chiropractic at Macquarie University.

Her experience of chiropractic whilst studying cemented her decision to become a chiropractor – her health was challenged and the chiropractic lifestyle transformed her from being lethargic and bedridden to driven and inspired.

Kathy first worked as a chiropractor in Toowoomba in Queensland, Australia before moving back home to set up her practice where she specialises in chiropractic care for women, pregnancy and children.

Kathy still enjoys skiing, rock climbing (although less so since the children) and the beach. When her hands are not busy working they are knitting, sewing or making something. She is married to the man of her dreams and they have two beautiful girls, Charlotte who is two and Eleanor, six months.

E: kathy@universalchiropractic.com.au
www.universalchiropractic.com.au

Sandy Clark

Sandy Clark B.Sc (Biol.Chem), B.App. Sc (Clinical Sc.), B Chiropractic Sc was born in Brisbane in the now closed Boothville hospital which, at the time, was as close to a natural active birth centre there was in Brisbane in 1969. As a child he grew up on the Sunshine Coast in Queensland, Australia where his daily life was body surfing with his family, riding bikes, skate boards and generally having great childhood adventures.

His first experience with Chiropractic was in 1980 when his parents took him for help with recurrent ear infections. After achieving a Bachelor of Science degree from Griffith University where he studied physics, cellular biology and biological chemistry, his many life-changing experiences through chiropractic adjustments naturally saw him return to university to study Chiropractic at the Royal Melbourne Institute of Technology. From 1998 until the present, he has practised in Brisbane and now owns and runs Grange Family Chiropractic where he specialises in SOT (Sacro-Occipital Technique) and NET (Neuro (body) Emotional (mind) Technique) adjusting. Sandy is also a certified Craniopath and for the last 10 years has studied Chiropractic Paediatrics, from specialist adjusting techniques and diagnostics to paediatric neurological development and assessment.

He is currently on the Board of the Chiropractors Association of Australia in Queensland and the Vice President of Sacro Occipital Technique Organisation of Australasia.

Grange Family Chiropractic
Cnr Blandford & Raymont Rds,
Grange Qld 4051

P: +61 (0)7 3356 8457
E: drsandy@grangefamilychiro.com.au
www.grangefamilychiro.com.au

Ed Groenhart BSc (Hons) MSc Doctor of Chiropractic – I came into Chiropractic after completing a Bachelor's degree in Physiology at the University of Newcastle upon Tyne. Having decided to use my new qualification as a springboard into a promising profession, I enrolled in the Master's Chiropractic course at the University of Surrey, Guildford. In 2001, after five and a half years' study, I was finally able to register as a chiropractor.

I am a member of the United Chiropractic Association, the British Chiropractic Sports Council, and have full registration in Australia as well as the UK. I have spent time working in practices around the south and east of England, as well as NSW, Australia.

I have special interests in Family and Sports Chiropractic and have worked at events all over Europe. It has been a pleasure helping elite athletes such as jockeys, triathletes and ice skaters achieve their goals.

My outside interests revolve around sports – I am a keen football player and enjoy running. I have run half-marathons, and the London and New York Marathons in 1999 and 2002 respectively. Naturally I receive chiropractic adjustments regularly as part of my healthy lifestyle.

I practise in the UK at Radcliffe Chiropractic Clinic.

---

www.rad-chiro.co.uk

Find me at uk.linkedin.com/pub/ed-groenhart/4/a83/419

Linda Balazic-Vandenberg

Linda Balazic-Vandenberg B. App. Sc. (Clinical Science/Chiropractic) is an Australian chiropractor. In 2002, she completed her chiropractic degree at RMIT in Melbourne and is currently in the final stages of completing her masters in Chiropractic Pediatrics at the University of Wales. She owns and runs a family practice in Hampstead in North London, UK. She has a passion for promoting a healthy lifestyle for families and utilises a gentle technique with babies and children to optimise their brain and neural development.

Natural Health Chiropractic
1st floor, 5a Heath St
Hampstead, London NW3 6TP

P: 0207 431 4882
E: lbalazic@hotmail.com
www.naturalhealthchiro.co.uk

Rachael Talbot DC, MSc, BSc – Following a successful career in the
Pharmaceutical Industry, Rachael retrained as a chiropractor, graduating
with First Class Honours from the Anglo European Chiropractic College,
Bournemouth, UK. Having grown three successful practices using traditional
biomechanical chiropractic techniques, Rachael now practices Network Spinal
Analysis and Somato Respiratory Integration. Both techniques are at the
forefront of the wellness movement and are forms of re-organizational healing.

Her practice, Chiropractic 4 Health, is the first of its kind in Wales, UK. Here
she is successfully pioneering this new approach, inspiring many to new levels
of health and wellbeing. She is amongst the first British chiropractors to be
recognised at the highest level within the worldwide Network Spinal Analysis
Community achieving Full Certification in the technique.

Aside from her busy practice, Rachael speaks regularly in the community and
makes time to train and mentor new chiropractors so they can experience the
great results she has seen and fulfil their potential.

She is passionate about caring for all ages from newborns to seniors.

---

www.chiropractic4health.co.uk

Paul McCrossin

Paul McCrossin B.App.Sci (Chiro) Chiropractor was born in Australia, training to be a Chiropractor at the Royal Melbourne Institute of Technology where he was on the student council. After graduating in 1995 he worked in various practices around Australia as a locum. He moved to the UK in 2000, settling in London. He has been involved politically in the profession as an executive member of the United Chiropractic Association (UCA) since 2001 and is presently head of the Peer and Ethics Committee assisting the membership in patient management. He has represented the UCA on various committees as the regulator in the UK of the General Chiropractic Council (GCC).

Paul is an avid skier and sportsman with an interest in running and triathlon, having completed eight marathons to date. He has had a role in the past as a chiropractor to members of the Canadian Biathlon team and for competitors in the Verbier Ride freestyle skiing competition. He has a family practice based in North London.

P: +44 20 8445 4355
E: finchley@bthcc.co.uk
www.finchleychiro.com

Carolyn Minster B. App. Sc. (Chiropractic) grew up in rural Victoria, Australia and started her working life there as a Registered Nurse. On completion of her nursing training she relocated to Melbourne and specialised in Neurosurgical nursing. She then went on to study Chiropractic at RMIT in Melbourne, graduating in 1992. She has since practised Chiropractic in Alice Springs, Sydney and at her current location in suburban Melbourne.

Carolyn and her husband Luke (also a chiropractor) have two sons aged 15 and 13, two daughters aged 10 and 7, a French exchange student and a slobbery Labrador.

Carolyn loves following her children's sports and reading – doesn't matter what it is. She is committed to local community and has served on the board of the Community Health Service, the Down Syndrome Association and her children's school committees.

She strongly believes that *every* body deserves Chiropractic, especially those bodies starting life with extra hurdles to overcome.

Chiropractic Life
1069 Doncaster Rd
Doncaster East, Vic 3109

P: +61 (0)3 9842 9255
E: Chirolife@optusnet.com.au

Matthew Doyle

Matthew Doyle MSc ACP Paed, BAppSc (Clinical), BChiroSc, BSc (Neurobiology) has been using regular chiropractic care since the early 1990s. As an avid sportsman, he played cricket to state schoolboy level and, more recently, has competed in the Scottish National Basketball League. The huge impact chiropractic has made on his improved recovery in sport, and the changes he saw in his family through chiropractic led to him following that path to become a chiropractor.

He gained his BSc in Neurobiology from the University of Queensland, and moved to Victoria to graduate with his BAppSc (Clinical), BChiroSc from RMIT University. Since moving to the UK in 2005 he has practised in England and Scotland. Due to his passion to help families and children, he completed the Anglo European College of Chiropractic's Master in Advanced Chiropractic Paediatric Practice in 2010 through Bournemouth University, and is currently practising in Glasgow, Scotland.

Glasgow Chiropractic
Level 3, St Vincent St
Glasgow, G3 6BY

P: 0141 222 2919
F: 0141 222 2918
E: drmatthewdoyle@gmail.com

Tracy Kennedy-Shanks

Tracy Kennedy-Shanks B.Sc. (Anatomy) D.C. USA comes from a long line of chiropractors. She is 4th generation with both her grandfather and great grandfather practising in Canada. Her father migrated to Australia as a chiropractor in the 1960s and started Kennedy Chiropractic Centre. It is now a large wellness-based family practice with 4 chiropractors.

Tracy graduated from Parker College in Dallas Texas, and moved back to Australia with her husband Glen in 1995. She is on the board of the Chiropractic Association of Australia as the regional representative for Queensland.

Kennedy Chiropractic Centre
130 Russell Street
Toowoomba Qld 4350
Australia
www.kennedychiro.com

Veronica Hope

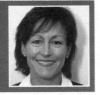

Veronica Hope B. App Sc. Chiropractic, Spinal Wellness Chiropractor, was born and raised in rural Victoria, Australia. As a young girl she witnessed firsthand the benefits of spinal adjustments and Chiropractic on the recovery from ill health of a family member. The impression from this experience was so profound that Veronica decided to become a chiropractor. She attended The Phillip Institute of Technology in Melbourne, Australia and graduated in 1990. She has completed extensive post graduate training in spinal care and holistic based healing. She is a respected and inspiring public speaker in the field of Wellness Chiropractic.

Veronica lives with her husband and two children in Kent in the UK where, in 1999, she established and continues to operate the Hope Spinal Wellness Centre. Having studied chiropractic and worked extensively in this field over the past twenty years, Veronica has a unique insight into how spinal and neurological dysfunction can affect the human health potential. She practises a Wellness Model and her purpose is to improve the health and wellbeing of the community through spinal and lifestyle adjustment.

E: hopechiro@yahoo.co.uk
www.hopespinalwellness.co.uk

Maryellen Stephens

Maryellen Stephens BScKIN, BScHumanSci (Chiro), MScChiro, MCC graduated from Dalhousie University in 1996, after studying Kinesiology. She worked with various sports teams and as a personal trainer before returning to college to study, graduating from the Anglo-European College of Chiropractic in 2000. Since then, Maryellen has embarked on many postgraduate courses in Pregnancy and Pediatrics, Craniopathy, and Neuro Emotional Technique, and is aiming to complete her MSc Clinical Chiropractic Pediatrics in due course.

Maryellen Stephens
Family Chiropractor
2 Alma Place, Redruth,
Cornwall TR15 2AT

P: 01209 219444

7 Church Street, Helston,
Cornwall TR13 8TA

P: 01326 560965
E: info@family-chiro.co.uk
www.family-chiro.co.uk

Robert Sandford

Rob Sandford Chiropractor BSc (hons), MSc (Chiro), DC was born in Plymouth and first visited a chiropractor at the age of four months. Having decided to become a chiropractor aged seven, Rob graduated from the Anglo-European College of Chiropractic in 2001 with a first class honours degree in human science and a Masters degree in Chiropractic.

After periods working in his home practice in Plymouth, London and Northern Ireland Rob settled back in Devon and opened Blue Mountain Family Chiropractic with his wife Melissa in 2003. In 2006 they opened a second office and now run two offices in the area, in Ashburton and Ivybridge.

Rob has two children with Melissa, as well as three stepchildren. All of the children have received chiropractic care throughout their lives and the family enjoys a chiropractic lifestyle.

Rob runs to keep fit and has completed three marathons and numerous half-marathons since 2007.

Blue Mountain Family Chiropractic
8 Erme Court
Leonards Road
Ivybridge, Devon PL21 0SZ

P: 01752 691118
E: bmfcivy@gmail.com

Blue Mountain Family Chiropractic
1st Floor Offices
11/13 North Street
Kings Bridge House
Ashburton, Devon TQ13 7QJ

P: 01364 654661
E: ashadmin@sandfordchiropractor.co.uk

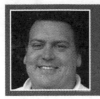

Roger Wood

Roger Wood M.Tech (Chiropractic), TPI-CGFI was born and educated in South Africa. After qualifying with a Masters Degree in Chiropractic, he decided to practise in England. In December 2005 he opened Innate Family Chiropractic Centre in Norwich, England.

Roger and his team strive to offer the highest standard of chiropractic care in a relaxed, caring and professional manner. He uses both manual and/or lighter, non manual, chiropractic techniques to improve spinal function, reduce nerve interference and help the body to regain and maintain optimal health. Roger is passionate about providing chiropractic care for the entire family and has a particular interest in providing care for the pregnant and paediatric patient, and in sports chiropractic.

Roger identifies that we have numerous options in healthcare and his goal is to increase awareness of what Chiropractic has to offer. He encourages the community to make informed decisions concerning their health and wellness.

Roger is a member of the United Chiropractic Association and registered with the General Chiropractic Council.

In 2008 he gained certification as a Golf Fitness Instructor with the Titleist Performance Institute (TPI).

Innate Family Chiropractic Centre
6 Clarence Road
Norwich NR1 1HH
England

www.innatechiro.co.uk

Robert Marin

Robert Marin B App Sc Chiropractic (RMIT), M.A.C.C, Dip Acup., graduated from RMIT University, Melbourne, Victoria in 1982. He is a Member of the Australasian College of Chiropractors. Rob has also done extensive training to further his skills including Relationship Training with Sondra Ray, Mental Emotional, Structural Analysis with Dr Lowell Ward DC, and Transactional Analysis with Ken Windes Game Academy. Dr Rob developed an interest in health education while studying 'Excellerated Learning' with Robert Kiyosaki and DC Cordoba.

In his practice in Hove, South Australia, Rob focuses on spine and nerve function repair with an emphasis on the correction and maintenance of lifestyle diseases brought on by lifestyle stresses. He has a special interest in chronic fatigue and poor energy. Education is a large part of the protocol with the patients as staying well is as important as getting well.

The Chiropractic Centre
371 Brighton Road
Hove SA 5048

P: +61 (0)8 8298 8711
E: heal@kern.com.au
W: Spinecheck.net

Mats Hansson

Mats Hansson DC, doctor of Chiropractic, runs a family wellness practice in Weymouth. His mission is to enhance the expression of vitality from within through chiropractic care and education.

Mats came across chiropractic at the age of eleven as an aspiring ice hockey player with a disability following a fall head first into the boards! He was unable to skate without experiencing a headache, palpitations and dizziness, so his mum took him to a chiropractor who, following an assessment, adjusted his first vertebra (C1) and, pronto, Mats was back in action, fully fit!

Having delivered his four children at home in water and raised them without any medical intervention (across-the-counter drugs included) or vaccinations – the chiropractic way – he is keen to educate parents about the amazing abilities their children have if left alone, fed well, exercised, and adjusted by a chiropractor.

Mats graduated from The Anglo European College of Chiropractic in Bournemouth in 1989 and has done postgraduate studies in pediatrics, cranial adjusting, sacral occipital technique (SOT), and applied kinesiology, neurolinguistic programming (NLP), nutrition and exercise applications/ evaluation.

He strongly believes in the commonsense ability of the people to wake up to the transparency of the medical model which does not respect the common laws of nature. Mats urges you to stop and ask yourself – does that make sense?

E: centre@hanssonchiropractic.co.uk

Kathy Rasch

Kathy Rasch B. App. Sc. (Chiropractic) – Born in Toowoomba, Queensland, Australia in June 1969, Kathy was inspired to pursue a career in Chiropractic having experienced the benefits first hand as a teenager. Graduating from Melbourne in 1991, Kathy and her partner Carl moved back to Toowoomba, practising as associates with Barham Chiropractic. In 1995 they settled in Maleny, fulfilling their dream of opening their own practice. Eight years and two beautiful daughters later, the family returned to Carl's home city, Melbourne, and settled in Mount Eliza. Kathy practised for 6 years at Lotus Chiropractic, with close friend Kimberlie Furness, specialising in pregnancy, birth and children.

At the end of 2008, Carl and Kathy created Wellbeing Natural Health Group, with centres in the Melbourne suburbs of Langwarrin and Mount Eliza. Kathy has also developed a Wellness Coaching program covering Nutrition, Exercise, Mind Power, Emotional Balance and Inner Connection.

Kathy and her family are committed to living a healthy lifestyle. In addition to practising in the Mount Eliza Wellbeing Centre, Kathy enjoys triathlons, running and personal training.

She is passionate about both caring for her patients on all levels and inspiring them to embrace greater health and wellbeing.

Wellbeing Natural Health Group
Mt.Eliza: Cnr. Wooralla Dr & Bundara Cres
P: +61 (0)3 9787 2111

Langwarrin: 96 Warrandyte Rd,
P: +61 (0)3 9785 6411

Mobiles:
Carl: +61 (0)422 385 490
Kathy: +61 (0)402 077 584

www.wellbeinggroup.com.au

Bruce Whittingham B.Sc(chiro) D.C. I spent the first eight years of my life thinking that everyone received chiropractic care all the time – the first floor of our home was my father's practice.

My siblings and I all became chiropractors because we shared the passion for helping to change lives in such a positive way. Having graduated from the Anglo-European College of Chiropractic (AECC) in Bournemouth, England, I travelled to Australia where I was introduced to kinesiology and sports chiropractic. I spent the next several years learning and developing my skills with chiropractors all over the world.

I have worked closely with various sporting organisations and teams and travelled with the Dick Johnson V8 motor racing team for the past four years, fine tuning the drivers whose bodies endure extreme ranges of physical stress whilst racing.

My current practice on the Gold Coast in Australia is full of people who enjoy being active and need to keep healthy to enjoy their lifestyle.

Surfers Paradise Chiropractic Centre
12 Thomas Drive, Chevron Island
Queensland, Australia

P: +61 (0)7 5539 9798
www.surfersparadisechiropractic.com.au

Monica Handa-Henshaw

Monica Handa-Henshaw BSc DC PgDip MCC FCBP – Chiropractor UK, who was born in Chiswick, London in 1970 was awarded a BSc Chiropractic (distinction) from Anglo European College of Chiropractic, Bournemouth, England in 1993 and holds numerous other post graduate qualifications including Pg Dip Clinical Chiropractic, Sacro-Occipital-Technique, Applied Kinesiology and CBP certification 1995.

Monica specialises in CBP (clinical biomechanics of posture) – the first female in the UK to gain certification in this technique. She also has interests in pregnancy and paediatrics, nutrition and sports injuries.

Her hobbies are exercising and reading when she isn't busy with husband Paul, an iron man who competes in marathons and triathlons (how handy to have a wife who's a chiropractor!), and their eight-year-old son Nikash and daughter Karina who is four. Both children have been adjusted regularly since their arrival in the world!

Monica owes her introduction to Chiropractic to her mother who had her youngest child after a gap of nearly nine years. Her health visitor advised her to see a chiropractor after she developed back pain and had tried all the usual avenues without any relief. As the chiropractor was very close to Monica's school, she would often meet her mum there. So began the journey towards Chiropractic. Her youngest brother is also now a chiropractor, working from the same office.

E: monica@optimumspine.com
www.optimumspine.com

Cathy Turnell BSc Hons, MChiro – Seeing the incredible effect that Chiropractic had on her parents was the reason that Cathy chose a career in Chiropractic. After graduating from Cardiff University with a BSc (Hons) in Biochemistry and Physiology she went on to study at the Anglo-European College of Chiropractic where she gained her Master of Chiropractic in 2006.

Cathy started out in practice as an associate gaining experience in two wellness-based chiropractic practices in the beautiful Lake District. She has relocated with her partner and is now working as an associate in Newcastle.

Centred Chiropractic
4 St James Terrace
Newcastle Upon Tyne
NE1 2NE

P: 0191 230 1777
www.newcastleupontynechiropractor.co.uk

References

Paula Moore Endnotes

1. NHS (the information centre for health and social care) www.ic.nhs.uk

2. Establishing a database of U.S. chiropractic health manpower data: furthering the development of research infrastructure.

   Smith M, Morschhauser S: Association for Health Services Research, Meeting. Abstr Book Assoc Health Serv Res Meet. 1999; 16; 426.

   Palmer Center for Chiropractic Research, Davenport, IA 52803, USA

3. Preamble to the Constitution of the World Health Organization as adopted by the International Health Conference, New York, 19–22 June, 1946; signed on 22 July 1946 by the representatives of 61 States (Official Records of the World Health Organization, no. 2, p. 100) and entered into force on 7 April 1948.

4. There are no hard and fast rules about transformation, which is what is so appealing about this approach to health. You *will* recognise your health transformation and how you recognise it will depend very much on how real your possibility is for you and that you continue to be *in action*. Transformation is not a destination but an ongoing process for your life.

Alan Scott References

1. Lopez AD, Mathers CD, Ezzati M, Jamison DT, Murray CJ (May 2006). "Global and regional burden of disease and risk factors, 2001: systematic analysis of population health data". Lancet 367 (9524): 1747–57.

2. Office of National Statistics (UK), Adult Psychiatric Morbidity in England, 2007: results of a household survey *Arch Gen Psychiatry*. 2005 Jun;62(6):593–602. Lifetime prevalence and age-of-onset distributions of DSM-IV disorders in the National Comorbidity Survey Replication.

   Kessler RC, Berglund P, Demler O, Jin R, Merikangas KR, Walters EE. Showed in USA up to 50% estimated life time rate of mental health issues)

John Swatland References

1. Quigley W. Heath M.S., D.C. Pioneering Mental Health: Institutional Psychiatric Care in Chiropractic. *Chiropractic History.*, Volume 3, Number1, 1983.

2. Williams NH, Hendry M, Lewis R, Russell I, Westmoreland A, Wilkinson C. Psychological response in spinal manipulation (PRISM): a systematic review of psychological outcomes in randomised controlled trials. *Complement Ther Med.* 2007 Dec; 15(4):271–83. Epub 2007 Mar 8.

3. Fawkes Carol. Psychological outcomes of spinal manipulation for low back pain: 2008 annual evidence update. *NHS Evidence - complementary and alternative medicine formerly a Specialist Library of the National Library for Health.* http://www.library.nhs.uk/cam/ViewResource.aspx?resID=294706

4. Kiecolt-Glaser JK, McGuire L, Robles TF, Glaser R Psychoneuroimmunology: psychological influences on immune function and health. *J Consult Clin Psychol,* 2002 Jun; 70(3):537–47. Also see neuropsychopharmacology article at: http://www.acnp.org/g4/gn401000069/ch069.html

5. Editorial. *British Journal of Psychiatry.* (2002) 180: 392-393.

6. Vernon HT, Dhami MS, Howley TP. Spinal manipulation and beta-endorphin: a controlled study of the effect of a spinal manipulation on plasma beta-endorphin levels in normal males. *J Manipulative Physiol Ther.* 1986 Jun; 9 (2):115.

7. Oh B, Butow P, Mullan B, Clarke S. Medical Qigong for cancer patients: pilot study of impact on quality of life, side effects of treatment and inflammation. *Am J Chin Med.* 2008;36(3):459–72.

8. Rousell Nathalie et al. Altered Breathing Patterns in Chronic Low Back Pain Patients. *European Spine Journal,* Volume 16, (pp 1066–1020.)

9. Seaman D, Winterstein J. Dysafferentation: a novel term to describe the neuropathophysiological effects of joint complex dysfunction. A look at likely mechanisms of symptom generation. *J Manipulative Physiol Ther.* 1998, 21 (4): 267–80.

10. Weil Andrew, Toms Michael. *Roots of Healing..* 1997. Hay House, (p2–3).

11. Doidge Norman. *The Brain That Changes Itself: Stories of Personal Triumph from the Frontiers of Brain Science..* 2007, Scribe. (p234).

12. Ibid. (p234)

13. Charlotte Leboeuf-Yde, DC, MPH, PhDa et al. Responses to Chiropractic Intervention: A Multination Survey *J Manipulative Physiol. Ther.* Volume 28, Issue 5, (pp 294–302) June 2005.

14. Pert, Candace, with Nancy Marriott. *Everything You Need to Know to Feel Go(o)d.* 2006, (p5), Hay House Inc.

15. Benson Herbert. *The Relaxation Response.* 1975, Avon Press.

16. Simonton O Carl, Simonton Stephanie Mathews, Creighton James L. *Getting Well Again.* 1992, Bantum.

17. Richard J. Davidson, PhD, Jon Kabat-Zinn, PhD. et al. Alterations in Brain and Immune Function Produced by Mindfulness Meditation *Psychosomatic Medicine.* 65:564–570 (2003)

18. Hanson Rick. *Buddha's Brain: the practical neuroscience of happiness, love and wisdom.* 2009, New Harbinger Publications. (p 85, cites studies by Davidson, Tang, Walsh and Shapiro).

19. Doidge, Norman, ibid, p43.

20. Interview with Richard Davidson Ph.D. © by Daniel Redwood D.C. (transcript). http://www.healthy.net/scr/interview.aspx?Id=306

21. Preventive Medicine Research Institute. Dr Ornish's non-profit institute website is at: http://www.pmri.org/research.html

Authors note: the complete list of references for this article numbered over fifty. The full list, along with web address links, will be available at the website www.hyperdomechiro.com.au.

Alan Brown References

1. Jan Hartvigsen, DC, PhD, and Lise Hestbaek, DC, PhD. 'Children and chiropractic care a window of opportunity'. *Journal of Manipulative Physiological Therapeutics 2009;* 32:603–605

2. Heisey, S. Richard Sc.D.; Adams, Thomas Ph.D.: 'Role of cranial bone mobility in cranial compliance'. *Neurosurgery 1993*, 33(5):869–876.

3. Sergueef N, Nelson KE, Glonek T. "The effect of cranial manipulation on the Traube-Hering-Mayer oscillation as measured by laser-Doppler flowmetry": *Alternative Therapies in Health and Medicine*.2002 Nov-Dec; 8(6):74–6

4. Jonathan Howat, M.P. *Chiropractic: Anatomy and Physiology of Sacro Occipital Technique.* Cranial Communication Systems, 14 Holyoake Road, Headington, Oxford OX3 8AE UK. 1999

5. *William Obstetrics* Chapter 18, vol 21 pages 436–437

6. Pistolese R.A. 'The Webster Technique: a chiropractic technique with obstetric implications'. *Journal of Manipulative and Physiological Therapeutics.* 2002 Jul–Aug; 25(6):E1–9.

7. Lise Hestbaek, PhD, Annette Jørgensen, DC, and Jan Hartvigsen, PhD: 'A description of children and adolescents in Danish chiropractic practice: results from a nationwide survey' *Journal of Manipulative and Physiological Therapeutics* 2009; 32:607–615

8. Biedermann Heiner MD. 'Manual therapy in children: Proposals for an etiologic model'. *Manipulative Physiological Therapeutics*; Volume 28 No 3. March/April 2005

9. Contribution of chiropractic therapy to resolving suboptimal breastfeeding: a case series of 114 infants', Joyce E. Miller, DC, Laura Miller, Ann-Kristin Sulesund, and Andriy Yevtushenkob. *Journal of Manipulative and Physiological Therapeutics* 2009; 32:670–674

10. Cheryl Hawk D.C. PhD. et al.*The Journal of Alternative and Complementary Medicine*. Volume 13, number 5, 2007, pp.491–512

11. Neils Nilsson DC M.D et al. 'The effect of spinal manipulation in the treatment of Cervicogenic headache'. *Journal of Manipulative and Physiological Therapeutics*. Vol 20, Number 5. June 1997

Sandy Clarke Colic Bibliography

1. 'Colic and disturbed sleep' Pluhar GR, Schubert PD; *Journal of Chiro Research and Clin Invest* 1991; 7(3):75–6

2. "Latent spinal cord and brain stem injury in newborn infants". Towbin A. *Develp Med Child Neurol* 1969; 11:54–68

3. 'Colic and Dysfunctional Nursing' Sheader, WE, *Journal of Clinical Chiropractic Paediatrics*, Vol. 4, No. 1, 1999.

4. 'Colic and Dysfunctional nursing' Cuhel JM, Powell M, *Journal of Clinical Chiropractic Pediatrics* Vol. 2, No. 2 1997. P. 150–154

5. *International Chiropractic Paediatric Association Newsletter*. May/June 1997. 'Gastrointestinal signs and symptoms of allergic diseases in children' Corvo M, Ghiglioni D, Gemellaro L, Sarratud T, Fiocchi A Pediatr Med Chir. 2009 Jul-Aug;31 (4):153–9

6. 'The crying infant: diagnostic testing and frequency of serious underlying disease'. Freedman SB, Al-Harthy N, Thull-Freedman J. *Pediatrics*. 2009 Mar;123(3):841–8

7. *J Nepal Med Assoc*. 2008 Oct-Dec; 47 (172):193–6. 'A study of abdominal pain in children'. Shakya KN, Dongol UM, Khadka SB

8. *World J Gastroenterol*. 2008 Aug 7; 14 (29):4662–6. 'Incidence and risk factors for infantile colic in Iranian infants'. Talachian E, Bidari A, Rezaie MH

9. 'Infantile colic incidence and associated risk factors: a cohort study' Saavedra MA, da Costa JS, Garcias G, Horta BL, Tomasi E, Mendonça R. *Pediatrics (Rio J)*. 2003 Mar-Apr; 79 (2):101–2.

10. *Arch Dis Child Fetal Neonatal* Ed. 2000 Jul;83 (1):F44–7. 'Fetal growth and infantile colic'. Søndergaard C, Skajaa E, Henriksen TB.

11. *J Dev Behav Pediatr.* 2002 Feb; 23 (1):1–8. 'Colicky infants according to maternal reports in telephone interviews and diaries: a large Scandinavian study'. Canivet C, Jakobsson I, Hagander B.

12. *Arch Dis Child Fetal Neonatal.* 2001 May; 84 (5):398–403. 'Systematic review of the occurrence of infantile colic in the community'. Lucassen PL, Assendelft WJ, van Eijk JT, Gubbels JW, Douwes AC, van Geldrop WJ.

13. *Pediatrics* 2004 Oct; 114(4):e497–505. 'Maternal smoking and infantile gastrointestinal dysregulation: the case of colic'. Shenassa ED, Brown MJ

14. *J Pediatr Health Care.* 1998 Sep-Oct; 2(5):256–62. 'New strategies for the treatment of colic: modifying the parent/infant interaction'. Dihigo SK.

15. *Pediatrics.* 2000 Jun; 105 (6):E84. 'Infant massage compared with crib vibrator in the treatment of colicky infants'. Huhtala V, Lehtonen L, Heinonen R, Korvenranta H

16. *J Pediatr Nurs.* 1989 Jun; 4(3):147–61. 'Colic: idiopathic, excessive, infant crying'. Pinyerd BJ, Zipf WB

17. *Child Care Health Development.* 2002 Sep; 28 (5):419–29. 'Excessively crying infant in the family: mother-infant, father-infant and mother-father interaction'. Räihä H, Lehtonen L, Huhtala V, Saleva K, Korvenranta H.

18. Hayden C, Mullinger B 'A preliminary assessment of the impact of cranial osteopathy for the relief of infantile colic. Complement Ther Clin Pract. 2006 May; 12 (2):83–90

19. J. Manipulative Physiol Ther. 2009 Oct, 32 (8):635–8. 'Long-term effects of infant colic: a survey comparison of chiropractic treatment and non-treatment groups'. Miller JE, Phillips HL.

20. 'Paternal depressive symptoms during pregnancy are related to excessive infant crying'. van den Berg MP, van der Ende J, Crijnen AA, Jaddoe VW, Moll HA, Mackenbach JP, Hofman A, Hengeveld MW, Tiemeier H, Verhulst FC. Clin Nurs. 2008 Jul; 17 (13):1754–61.

21. 'Effectiveness of massage, sucrose solution, herbal tea or hydrolysed formula in the treatment of infantile colic'. Arikan D, Alp H, Gözüm S, Orbak Z, Cifçi EK. J Clin Nurs. 2008 Nov; 17 (21):2945-7; discussion 2947–8)

22. Towben study 1969

Linda Balazic-Vandenberg References

1. Meeker W C, Haldeman S 'Chiropractic: A profession at the crossroads of mainstream and alternative medicine'. Ann Intern Med. 2002; 136:216–227.

2. Arnig Howe A 1994 'Scientific ramifications for providing prenatal and neonatal chiropractic care'. *Chiropractic Pediatrics.* Vol 1 No 2. August

3. French L M, Dietz F R 1999 'Screening for developmental Dysplasia of the hip'. *Am Fam Physician* 60. July: 177–188.

4. Davies N J 2000 *Chiropractic Pediatrics: A clinical handbook*. Churchill Livingstone, Edinburgh

5. Biedermann H 2005 *Manual therapy in children for an etiologic model*. JMPT, 28(6):460

6. Lewit K Barth J A Leipzig 'Functional Disorders of the spine in children'. *Manuelle Therapie*. 1973; 2(7):50–54)

7. Hannon S M. 'Objective Physiologic Changes and Associated Health Benefits of Chiropractic Adjustments in Asymptomatic Subjects: A review of the literature'. JVSR 2004. (pg 1–9)

   http://www.jvsr.com/abstracts/index.asp?id=201

8. Van Breda, WM, Juan M. 'A comparative study of the health status of children raised under the health care models of chiropractic and allopathic medicine'. *Journal of Chiropractic Research* 5 (Summer):101–103, 1989.

9. Davies N J 2000 *Chiropractic Pediatrics: A clinical handbook*.

   Churchill Livingstone, Edinburgh

10. Abram, N. *The Chiropractic Report*. July 1992 Vol. 6 No. 5.

    Bourdillon JE, Day EA, Bookhout MR: 'Spinal Manipulation', 5th edition. Oxford, England, Butterworth-Heinemann Ltd, 1992.

11. Barham-Floreani J 2009. *Well Adjusted Babies*. Vitality Productions Pty Ltd, Australia.

12. 'Proceedings of the 1991 International Conference on Spinal Manipulation', FCER; 227–229 Shambaugh P, Pearlman RC, Hauck K

    sourced by Maginness G 2001. C4K 'Chiropractic for kids'. Paediatric Research CD ROM. Available.http://www.c4k.com.au

13. Carrick F R. 1997. 'Changes in brain function after manipulation of the cervical spine.' JMPT Oct; 20(8) pp529–45.

Rachael Talbot References

1. Comorbidity of Dyslexia, Dyspraxia, Attention Deficit Disorder (ADD), Attention Deficit Hyperactive Disorder (ADHD), Obsessive Compulsive Disorder (OCD) and Tourette's Syndrome in Children: Pauc, R. A Prospective Epidemiological Study. Clinical Chiropractic 2005 (Dec); 8(4) 189–198.

2. An evaluation of chiropractic manipulation as a treatment of hyperactivity in children. Giesen JM, Center DB, leach RA J Manipulative Physiol Ther 1989 (Oct);12 (5):353–363

3. Improvement in Attention in Patients Undergoing Network Spinal Analysis: A Case Series Using Objective Measures of Attention. Pauli Y. Journal of Vertebral Subluxation Research, August 23,2007; 1–9

4. Bastecki AV, Harrison DE, Haas JW. Cervical kyphosis is a possible link to attention-deficit/hyperactivity disorder. J Manipulative Physiol Ther. 20040ct;27(8):e14.

5. Lovett l, Blum Cl Behavioral and Learning Changes Secondary to Chiropractic Care to Reduce Subluxations in a Child with Attention Deficit Hyperactivity Disorder: A Case Study *Journal of Vertebral Subluxation Research* Oct 2006: 1–6.

6. International Chiropractic Pediatric Association Newsletter, May/June 1997

7. The effect of chiropractic treatment on students with learning and behavioral impairments resulting from neurological dysfunction (part 1). Brzozowske WT, Walton EV. J. *Aust Chiro Assoc* 1980;11(7):13–18. and Part II: J. *Aust Chiro Assoc* 1980;11(8):11–17.

8. ADHD – A multiple case study. Wendel P, *International Chiropractic Pediatric Association*. March/April 1998.

9. Case study: the effect of utilizing spinal manipulation and craniosacral therapy as the treatment approach for attention deficit-hyperactivity disorder. Phillips CJ. *Proceedings on the National Conference on Chiropractic and Pediatrics* (ICA), 1991:57–74.

10. Effects of biomechanical insult correction on attention deficit disorder. Arme J. *J of Chiropractic Case Reports*, Vol. 1 No.1 Jan. 1993

11. EEG and CEEG studies before and after upper cervical or SOT category 11 adjustment in children after head trauma, in epilepsy, and in "hyperactivity." Hospers LA, V *Proc of the National Conference on Chiropractic and Pediatrics* (ICA) 1992;84–139.

12. Blum Cl, Cuthbert 5, Williams 5, Developmental Delay Syndromes and Chiropractic: A Case Report. *International Conference on Chiropractic Research*. Vilamoura, Portugal – May 17–19, 2007: CM53.

13. Passingham, R.E. (1975). Changes in the size and organization of the brain in man and his ancesteors. Brain, Behaviour and Evolution. 11, 73–90

14. The Relationship between Convergence Insufficiency and ADHD. Strabismus 2005 Dec;13(4):163–8. David B. Granet, MD FACS FAAO FAAP, Cintia F. Gomi MD, Ricardo Ventura, MD, Andrea Miller-Scholte, CO

15. Levin et al. (1987). Magnetic resonance imaging and computerized tomography in relation to the neurobehavioral sequelae of mild and moderate head injuries. Journal of Neurosurgery, 66, 706–713.

16. Blumer, D., & Benson, D. Personality changes with frontal and temporal lobe lesions. In D. Benson and D. Blumer, eds. Psychiatric Aspects of Neurologic Disease. New York: Grune & Stratton, 1975.

17. Melillo R, Leisman G, *Neurobehavioural Disorders of Childhood. An Evolutionary Perspective*. Kluwer Academic/Plenum Publishers, New York 2004

18. Functional Magnetic Resonance Imaging: About the Cover (cover picture) Journal of Vertebral Subluxation Research, 1998; 2(1): Cover

19. Pert. C, Chopra. D. *Molecules of Emotion: Why you Feel the Way you Feel*. Pocket Books (1999)

20. A Retrospective Assessment of Network Care Using a Survey of Self-Rated Health, Wellness and Quality of Life. Blanks RH, Schuster TL, Dobson M. Journal of Vertebral Subluxation Research, 1997; 1(4): 15–31

Paul McCrossin – Backpack Suppliers

UNITED KINGDOM

Marathon School Supplies Ltd
+44 01932 567 700
www.marathonss.com
sales@marathonss.com

AUSTRALIA

Spartan School Supplies
Free call 1800 815 557
info@spartanss.com.au
www.spartanss.com.au

NEW ZEALAND

Chiropak® available from
Park Lane Handbags Ltd
PO Box 7267
Sydenham
Christchurch NZ 8002
(64) 3366 5172
(64) 3365 4015

Matthew Doyle References

1. Fysh, Peter. Chronic recurrent otitis media: case series of five patients with recommendations for case management. *J Clin Chiro Ped*. 1996, Vol. 1(2), 66–78.

2. Peet, J. Case study: chiropractic results with child with recurring otitis media accompnaied by effusion. *Chiropractic Pediatrics*. 1996, Vol. 2, 8–10.

3. Phillips, N. Vertebral Subluxation and otitis media: a case study. J *Chiro Res Clin Inv*. 1992, Vol. 8, 38–39.

4. Thomas, D. Irritable child with chronic ear effusion/infections responds to chiropractcic care. *Chiropr Ped*. 1997, Vol. 3, 13–14.

5. Fallon, JM. The role of the chiropractic adjustment in the care and treatment of 332 children with otitis media. *J Clin Chiro Ped*. 1997, Vol. 2, 167–183.

6. Froehle, RM. Ear Infection: a retrospective study examining improvement from chiropractic care and analyzing for influencing factors. *JMPT*. 1996, Vol. 19, 169–177.

7. Sawyer, CE., Evans, RL., Boline PD., et al. A feasibility study for chiropractic spinal manipulation versus sham spinal manipulation from chronic otitis media with effusion in children. *JMPT*. 1999, Vol. 22, 292–298.

8. Saunders, L. Chiropractic treatment of otitis media with effusion: a case report and literature review of the epideiological risk factors that predispose towards the condition and that influence the outcome of chiropractic treatment. *Clin Chiro*. 2004, Vol. 7, 168–173.

9. Vallone, S., Fallon, J. Treatment protocols for the chiropractic care of common pediatric conditions: otitis media and asthma. *J Clin Chiro Ped*. 2007, Vol. 2(1), 113–115.

10. Mills, MV., Henley, CE., Barnes, LL., et al. The use of osteopathic manipulative treatment as adjuvant therapy in children with recurrent acute otitis media. *Arch Ped Adol Med*. 2003, Vol. 157, 861–866.

11. Zhang, J., Synder, B. Effect of the Toftness chiropractic adjustments for children with acute otitis media. *J Vertebral Subluxation Re*s. 2004, Vol. March 29, 1–4.

12. Palmer, DD. *Textbook of the Science, Art and Philosophy of Chiropractic. Portland*, Oregan : Portland Printing House Company, 1910.

13. Legros, J., Hitoto, H., Garnier, F., et al. Clinical qualitative evaluation of the diagnosis of acute otitis media in general practice. *Int J Ped Otorh*. 2008, Vol. 23(5), 392–399.

14. Jesenaki, M., Rennerova, Z., Babusikova, E., et al. Food Allergens and respiratory symptoms. *J Phys & Pharm*. 2008, Vol. 59(6), 311–320.

15. Vergison, A., Dagan, R., Arguedas, A., et al. Otitis media and its consequences: beyond the earache. *Lancet Inf Dis*. 2010, Vol. 10(3), 195–203.

16. Maxwell, PR., Rink, E., Kumar, D., Mendall, MA. Antibiotics increase functional abdominal symptoms. *Am J Gastroenterol*. 2002, Vol. 97(1), 104–108.

17. Keith, T., Saxena, S., Murray, J., Sharland, M. Risk benefit analysis of restricting antimicrobial prescribing in children: what do we really know? *Curr Opin Inf Dis*. 2010, Vol. April 6, Epub ahead of print.

18. Moro, ML., Marchi, M., Gagliotti, C., et al. Why do pediatricians prescribe antibiotics? Results of an italian regional project. *BMC Pediatrics*. 2009, Vol. 9, 69.

19. Physcians, American Academy of Pediatrics and American Academy of Family. Clinical Practice Guidelines – diagnosis and management of acute otitis media. *Pediatrics*. 2004, Vol. 113(5), 1451–1465.

20. Lous, J., Burton, M., Ovesen, T., et al. Grommets (ventilation tubes) for hearing loss

associated wiht otitis media with effusion in children. *Cochrane Database fo Systematic Reviews*. Vol. Issue 1, Art. No.: CD001801. DOI: 10.1002/14651858.CD001801.pub2.

21. Miller, J., Benfield, K. Adverse effects of spinal manipulative therapy in children younger than 3 years: a retrospective study in a chiropractic teaching clinic. *JMPT*. 2008, Vol. 31, 419–423.

22. Alacantara, J., Ohm, J., Kunz, D. The safety and effectiveness of pediatric chiropractic: a survey of chiropractors and parents in a practice based research network. *Explore*. 2009, Vol. 5 , 290–295.

23. Vohra, S., Johnston, B., Cramer, K., Humphreys, K. Adverse events associated with pediatric spinal manipulation: a systematic review. *Pediatrics*. 2007, Vol. 119, e275–e283.

24. Gotlib, A., Rupert, R. Chiropractic manipulation in pediatric health conditions - an updated systematic review. *Chiro & Osteo*. 2008, Vol. 16(11), doi:10.1186/1746-1340-16-11.

25. Hawk, C., Khorsan, R., Lisi, AJ., et al. Chiropractic Care for nonmusculoskeletal conditions: a systematic review with implications for whole systems research. *J Alt & Comp Med*. 2007, Vol. 13(5), 491–512.

26. Cramer, G., Budgell, B., Henderson, C., et al. Basic science research related to chiropractic spinal adjusting: the state of the art and recommendations revisited. *JMPT*. 2006, Vol. 29(9), 726–761.

27. Subbarrao, P., Mandhane, PJ., Sears, M. Asthma:epidemiology, etiology and risk factors. *CMAJ*. 2009, Vol. 181(9), e181–e190.

Rob Sandford – Asthma References

1. 'Pulmonary Disorders: Asthma'. R. Blair, J.S. Breit, S. P. Peters. *Merck Manual Professional Edition*. April 2008. http://www.merck.com/mmpe/sec05/ch048/ch048a.html

2. 'Where do we stand? Asthma in the UK today'. *Asthma UK*. 2006 www.asthma.org.uk

3. 'Asthma'. C. H. Fanta. *New England Journal of Medicine*, 360:1002-1014, March 5, 2009

4. 'Trends in Childhood asthma: Prevalence, Health care utilization and Mortality'. L. J. Akinbami, MD. *Pediatrics* Vol. 110 No. 2 August 2002. Pp315–322

5. 'Asthma and other wheezing disorders in children'. D. Keeley, and M. McKean. *Clinical Evidence. BMJ Publishing Group Ltd*. 2006.

6. 'Changes in asthma prevalence: two surveys 15 years apart'. M. L. Burr, B. K. Butland, S King, E Vaughan Williams. *Archives of Disease in Children* 1989; 64: 1452–1456

7. 'Comparison of regularly scheduled with as-needed use of albuterol in mild asthma'. J.M. Drazen, E. Israel, H.A. Boushey, V.M. Chinchilli, J.V. Fahy, J.E. Fish, S.C. Lazarus, R.F. Lemanske, R.J. Martin, S.P. Peters, C. Sorkness, S.J. Szefler. *New England Journal of Medicine* 1996; 335:841–7

8. 'Long-term effects of a long-acting beta 2-adrenoceptor agonist, salmeterol, on airway hyperresponsiveness in patients with mild asthma'. D. Cheung, M.C. Timmers, A.H. Zwinderman, E.H. Bel, J.H. Dijkman, P.J. Sterk. *New England Journal of Medicine* 1992; 327(17):1198–203

9. 'The use of beta-agonists and the risk of death and near death from asthma. W.O. Spitzer, S. Suissa, P. Ernst, R.I. Horwitz, B. Habbick, D. Cockcroft, J.F. Boivin, M. McNutt, A.S. Buist, A.S. Rebuck. *New England Journal of Medicine* 1992; 326:501–6

10. 'The effect of regular inhaled albuterol on exercise-induced bronchoconstriction'. M.D. Inman, P.M. O'Byrne. *American Journal of Respiratory and Critical Care Medicine* 1996; 153:65–9

11. 'Regular inhaled beta-agonist treatment in bronchial asthma'. M.R. Sears, D.R. Taylor, C.G. Print, D.C. Lake, Q.Q. Li, E.M. Flannery, D.M. Yates, M.K. Lucas, G.P. Herbison. *Lancet* 1990; 336:1391–6

12. 'Bronchodilator treatment in moderate asthma or chronic bronchitis: continuous or on demand? A randomised controlled study'. C.P. van Schayck, E. Dompeling, C.L. van Herwaarden, H. Folgering, A.L. Verbeek, H.J van der Hoogen, C. van Weel. *British Medical Journal* 1991; 303:1426–31

13. 'Dexamethasone in bronchiolitis: a randomised controlled trial'. G. Roosevelt, K. Sheehan, J. Grupp-Phelan, R.R. Tanz, R. Listernick. *Lancet* 1996; 348(9023):292–5

14. 'Dexamethasone in salbutamol-treated inpatients with acute bronchiolitis: a randomized, controlled trial'. T.P. Klassen, T. Sutcliffe, L.K. Watters, G.A. Wells, U.D. Allen, M.M. Li. *Journal of Pediatrics* 1997; 130(2):191–6

15. 'Lung function in relation to thoracic spinal mobility and kyphosis'. Mellin , R. Harjula. *Scandinavian Journal of Rehabilitation Medicine* 1987; 19(2):89–92

16. 'Specific upper cervical chiropractic care and lung function'. R. Kessinger. *Canadian Respiratory Journal* 1997; 4(1): 27

17. 'Changes in pulmonary function associated with upper cervical specific chiropractic care'. R. Kessinger. *Journal of Vertebral Subluxation Research* 1997; 1(3): 43–9

18. 'Chiropractic and lung volumes - A retrospective study'. C. Masarsky, M. Weber. *American Chiropractic Association Journal of Chiropractic* 1986; 23(9): 65–8

19. 'A comparison of the effect of chiropractic treatment on respiratory function in patients with respiratory distress symptoms and patients without'. C. Hviid. *Bull Eur Chiro Union* 1978; 26: 17–34

20. 'Chronic asthma and chiropractic spinal manipulation: a randomized clinical trial'. N.H. Nielsen, G. Bronfort, T. Bendix, F. Madsen, B. Weeke. *Clinical and Experimental Allergy* 1995; 25 (1): 80–88

21. 'Asthma in a chiropractic clinic: a pilot study'. J.R. Jamison, K. Leskovic, S. Lepore, P. Hannon. *Journal of the Australian Chiropractic Association* 1986; 16(4):137–43

22. 'Prognostic factors in bronchial asthma in chiropractic practice'. N. Nilsson, B. Christainson. *Journal of the Australian Chiropractic Association* 1988; 18(3):85–7

23. 'Contact between preschool children with chronic diseases and the authorized health services and forms of alternative therapy'. B. Vange. *Ugeskr Laeger* 1989; 151(28):1815–8

24. 'An impairment rating analysis of asthmatic children under chiropractic care'. R.L. Graham, R.A. Pistolese. *Journal of Vertebral Subluxation Research* 1997; 1(4): 41–8

25. 'Chronic pediatric asthma and chiropractic spinal manipulation: A prospective clinical series and randomized clinical pilot study'. G. Bronfort, R.L. Evans, P. Kubic, P. Filkin. *Journal of Manipulative and Physiological Therapeutics* 2001; 24(6): 369–77

26. 'Chiropractic management of 47 asthma cases'. W.C Amalu. *Today's Chiropractic* Vol. 29 No. 6 November/December 2000

Rob Sandford – Arthritis References

1. 'About Arthritis. *Arthritis Care*. www.arthritiscare.org.uk/AboutArthritis.

2. 'Estimates of the prevalence of arthritis and other rheumatic conditions in the United States: Part II' C. Helmick, D. Felson, R.C. Lawrence, S. Gabriel, R. Hirsch, C.K. Kwoh, M.H. Liang, H.M. Kremers, M.D. Mayes, P .A. Merkel, S.R. Pillemer, J.D. Reveille, J.H. Stone, *Arthritis & Rheumatism*. Volume 58 Issue 1, Pages 15 – 25. Published Online: 28 Dec 2007

3. 'Estimates of the prevalence of arthritis and other rheumatic conditions in the United States: Part II'. R.C. Lawrence, D.T. Felson, C.G. Helmick, L.M. Arnold, H. Choi, R .A. Deyo, S. Gabriel, R. Hirsch, M.C. Hochberg, G.G. Hunder, J.M. Jordan, J. N. Katz, H.M. Kremers, F. Wolfe. *Arthritis & Rheumatism*.Volume 58 Issue 1, Pages 26 – 35. Published Online: 28 Dec 2007

4. 'Arthritis Information: Osteoarthritis' *Arthritis Research UK*. www. arthritisresearchuk. org/arthritis_information/arthritis_types__symptoms/osteoarthritis.aspx#non

5. 'Etiopathogenesis of Osteoarthritis'. K.D. Brandt,; P. Dieppe; E. Radin. *Medical Clinics of North America* 2008. 93 (1): 1–24.

6. 'Osteoarthritis – National clinical guideline for care and management in adults'. P. Conaghan. National Institute for Health and Clinical Excellence. http://www.nice.org.uk/nicemedia/pdf/CG059FullGuideline.pdf

7. 'Understanding NSAIDs: from aspirin to COX-2'. G.A. Green. *Clinical Cornerstone* 2001 3 (5): 50–60.

8. 'Experimental Models of osteoarthritis: the role of immobilization'. T. Videman. *Clinical Biomechanics*. 1987; 2:223–229.

9. 'Rheumatoid arthritis, a case report'. W. Nelson. *Chiropractic Technique* 1990; 2:17–19.

10. 'Disc regeneration: reversibility is possible in spinal osteoarthritis'. O.J. Ressel.

International Chiropractors Association Review March/April 1989 pp. 39–61.

11. 'Osteoarthritis, chiropractic, and nutrition: osteoarthritis considered as a natural part of a three stage subluxation complex: its reversibility: its relevance and treatability by chiropractic and nutritional correlates'. D.L. Berkson *Medical Hypotheses* 1991 Dec; 36(4):356–67.

12. 'Osteoarthritis: a review of the cell biology involved and evidence for reversibility'. J.H. Bland, S.M. Cooper, S. E. M. Cooper. *Arthritis and Rheumatism* 14 (2): 106–133, 1984.

13. 'The reversibility of osteoarthritis.' J.H. Bland. *American Journal of Medicine*, 75:16–26, 1983.

14. 'Use of complementary therapies for arthritis among patients of rheumatologists'. J.K. Rao, K. Mihaliak, K. Kroenke, J. Bradley, W.M. Tierney, M. Weinberger. *Annals of Internal Medicine* 1999; 131:409–416.

Monica Handa References

1. www.acatoday.org/pdf/PDR/ChiropracticTechniques.pdf

2. www.drzemelka.com/thompson.htm

3. Fuhr, Arlan W.; J. Michael Menke (February 2005). "Status of Activator Methods Chiropractic Technique, Theory, and Practice". *Journal of Manipulative and Physiological Therapeutics* 28 (2): e1–e20.

4. Subject: Activator Methods Chiropractic Technique: General Articles

   Title: The Activator Story: Development of a New Concept in Chiropractic.

   Reference: Dennis M. Richards...Chiropractic Journal of Australia March 1994 (Mar); 24(1): pp.28–32

5. www.ncbi.nlm.nih.gov › ... › J Chiropr Med › v.2(1); Winter 2003

6. Getzoff H, Sacro Occipital Technique (SOT): A Method of Chiropractic *Proceedings of Pathways to Success – Credentialing and Technique Validity*: Assessing the Comparative Validity of Chiropractic Techniques, Jun 1996: 1–4.

7. www.chirobase.org/05RB/BCC/11d.html

8. www.logan.edu/SubPages.aspx?pID=27&mhID=148&splpID=5

9. www.coxtechnic.com

10. www.idealspine.com

11. http://www.chiro.org/ChiroZine/pierce.shtml

12. www.motionpalpation.org

13. www.appliedkinesiology.com

14. www.atlasorthogonality.com

15. Position paper for orthogonally-based upper cervical chiropractic care by Kirk Eriksen, D.C.

16. www.nucca.org

17. www.pettibonsystem.com

18. www.orthospinology.org

Cathy Turnell References

1. Batmanghelidj. F, (2000), *Your Body's Many Cries For Water*, The Tagman Press.

2. Booth. F.W., Chakravarthy. M.V., Gordon. S.E., Spangenburg. E.E. (2002), 'Waging war on physical inactivity: using modern molecular ammunition against an ancient enemy'. *Journal of Applied Physiology*, 93 (1): 3–30.

3. Cordain. L., Gotshall. R.W., Eaton. S.B., Eaton. S.B. 3rd. (1998). 'Physical activity, energy expenditure and fitness: an evolutionary perspective'. *International Journal of Sports Medicine* 19 (5): 328–335.

4. Eaton. S.B., Cordain. L., Lindenburg. S. (2002), 'Evolutionary health promotion: a consideration of common counterarguments'. *Preventative Medicine* 34 (2): 119–123.

5. Rubin. C.T. McLeod, K.T., Bain. S.D. (1990), 'Functional strains and cortical bone adaptation: epigenetic assurance of skeletal integrity'. *Journal of Biomechanics*, 23; 1: 43–54.

6. Morningstar, M.W., Pettobin, B.R., Schlappi, H., Schlappi, M., Ireland, T.V. (2005), 'Reflex control of the spine and posture: a review of the literature from a chiropractic perspective'. *Chiropractic and Osteopathy*, 13 (16) 1–17.

7. Ruff. C., Holt. B., Ttrinkaus. E. (2006), 'Who's afraid of the big bad Wolff?: Wolff's Law and bone functional adaptation'. *American Journal of Physical Anthropology*, 129 (4): 484–498.

8. Troyanovich, S.J., Harrison, D.E., Harrison, D.D. (1998). 'Structural rehabilitation of the spine and posture: Rationale for treatment beyond the resolution of symptoms'. *Journal of Manipulative and Physiological Therapeutics*, 21 (1), 37–50.

9. Videman, T. (1987) 'Experimental models of osteoarthritis: the role of immobilization'. *Clinical Biomechanics*, 2, 223–229.

Epilogue and Thanks

By Cyndi O'Meara

Dr John Demartini, chiropractor and philosopher, said: "The greatest art form that exists on this planet is the human body – a magnificently structured temple of sacred architecture ... Many people spend a great deal of time in front of the mirror focusing on what they perceive as imperfections of their body rather than focusing on its magnificently balanced perfection. Being grateful for your body and for the multitude of its powerful gifts can make the difference between experiencing wellness or illness in your life."

We are given just one body in our life but we fail to love it, fuel it with foods it has evolved to eat and maintain it with structural tuning. Most people take better care of their cars, making sure only the right fuel goes into it and that it is tuned and balanced every 10,000 km or so. The sad thing is that you can have as many cars as you can afford in your life but you can only have one body. Your body needs to be nourished and structurally tuned and loved in order for it to take you through your entire life with energy, vitality and health.

Chiropractic care, good nutrition, rest and relaxation, hydration with pure water, and a good positive attitude about life and the world is what has got me through with vibrant health. I have been associated with the chiropractic profession all my life and felt that the philosophy of this magnificent healing art was not being made available to the public in its entirety, so I decided to find chiropractors who were keen to spread the word about the benefits of maintaining structure and integrity in the body, and this is how this book came about. I wanted this book for the public, who mainly had the belief that health comes from an outside source rather than an inside force. Chiropractors and my type of eating regime never claim to cure anything. What we claim is that when the body (and mind) is well nourished and structurally aligned, it will function at a greater energy and heal itself. Welcome to abundant health!

This book could not have been possible without the input from many people. Firstly I want to thank Chen Tay an amazing, inspirational chiropractor and mentor who first suggested I do this project. Thank you to Sarah Farrant for your fabulous input. Thank you to Carla Francis who made sure all the authors were organised and on time with their information. Thank you to Suzanne Dean who has worked with each author to tell their story with passion, love and understanding. Thank you to Holly Odgers for making these pages come to life with her stunning layouts. And last but not least, thank you to each of the authors who saw the same vision I had to educate the public about how chiropractic changes lives.

Cyndi O'Meara
Nutritionist, Lifestylist and Chiropractic Advocate